WHAT TO DO *RIGHT NOW*
(and later today, tomorrow, and next week)

WHEN YOUR CHILD IS SUICIDAL

"Tara's book is a quick read which provides you with the nitty gritty details you need to know NOW to take care of your kid, your family and yourself when you have a child who is struggling with suicidal thoughts and behaviors. She navigates this challenging subject with grounded advice based on her own experience as well as compassion and hope. I would feel comfortable recommending this to the families and loved ones of any patient I am caring for. It is a great resource."

—INGA GISKE, DNP, PMHNP-BC
Consultation Liaison Psychiatry

"This was the book I needed when my child was in crisis and attending college over 2000 miles from home. Tara has written a step-by-step guide to help not only your child or young adult, but also yourself in the midst of a parent's worst nightmare. I hope and pray you don't need this book, but if you do, I am grateful she has written it."

—KATHRYN R., parent

"In an approachable and heartfelt manner, Tara says everything I wish families could know about the journey of a young person's mental health crisis. This book will certainly be a trusted companion for many caregivers, providing both concrete tips and tools, but also the solace of knowing they are not alone on this path."

—NAOMI FISHMAN, MD
Board Certified Child and Adolescent Psychiatrist

"Facing suicide is scary for everyone involved, but Tara Rolstad's **What to do RIGHT NOW** is a honest and complete book that gives parents tools, tips and suggestions from someone who has been there. Based on research and clinical theory as well as personal experience, it's a great guide for parents written in real-life language on real-life situations."

—ELIZABETH MCERLEAN, LCSW, LISW

"I think this book will be a great resource for parents new to having a child with mental illness. I remember the first time my child, then 14 years old, told me she wanted to kill herself. We went to the ER and she was placed under a Baker Act. I had no idea what I was supposed to do once I drove away from the hospital without her. This book would have helped a lot."

—LEIGH ANN, parent

WHAT TO DO *RIGHT NOW*

(and later today, tomorrow, and next week)

WHEN YOUR CHILD IS SUICIDAL

TARA ROLSTAD

Paperback ISBN: 979-8-9925477-0-2

TTTM Publishing

Important Disclaimers

This book is not medical advice, and the author is a layperson, not a medical or mental health provider of any kind.

The advice herein is not intended to replace the services of trained health professionals or be a substitute for medical advice. You are advised to consult with your health care professional with regard to matters relating to your health and that of your child, and, in particular, regarding matters that may require diagnosis or medical attention. Never rely on the information in this book to the exclusion of your medical team.

Please note: IF YOUR CHILD HAS A SERIOUS MENTAL ILLNESS SUCH AS BIPOLAR DISORDER, SCHIZOPHRENIA OR SCHIZO-AFFECTIVE DISORDER, they may have a specific symptom called anosognosia, or lack of insight. Anosognosia means that your child literally does not, and cannot, see that they are ill. *They do not have insight.* When a person without insight is actively suicidal, they need close supervision and immediate medical care, as this is a situation that cannot be handled at home. In that situation the recommendations in this book may not be appropriate. Remember, never rely on the information in this book to the exclusion of your medical team.

This book is dedicated to the young people I've loved who sometimes didn't want to live, who are stronger and more courageous than I will ever have to be; and to my bonus mom, Edde Rolstad, without question the Best Mother-in-Law on the Planet, who helped me get this book over the finish line.

Contents

Author's Note

This book is for you if your child or teen is suicidal. That's relatively straightforward, yes? It is particularly for you if the hospital just discharged your child to you; or if the hospital won't admit your child because they aren't deemed to be at *quite* enough risk; or they are having suicidal thoughts, but it isn't quite necessary to go to the hospital, yet you still have to get through this afternoon, and tomorrow, and next Tuesday, and **no one will tell you what to actually DO.**

It is also for you if your child isn't suicidal today, but they were recently, or they live with frequent suicidal thoughts, or you are concerned that may happen. This book is for you if you are the parent, caregiver, grandma or grandpa, auntie or uncle, close family friend, or you love a young person who lives with suicidal thoughts or serious mental health issues. *(Also, though I wrote this book primarily for parents and caregivers of kids college-age and younger, much of it may be helpful if you are a parent of a young adult or adult child.)*

I have been where you are, or at least I've been somewhere that looks a lot like where you are. I have actually been there relatively recently, a couple of times.

In fact, I've struggled a little bit, feeling like maybe I shouldn't write this book, or publish this book, because what if . . .? What if the young people I love who have lived with suicidal thoughts . . . well, you know. What if they actually die by suicide?

But if I wait until I'm sure those I love are totally well, and I'm one hundred percent sure it's "safe" to share this with you, then you will continue to feel just as alone as I have felt, as every parent or caregiver feels when they can't find any help or information on how to do this impossible thing: to walk alongside a young person who feels like they want to die.

No one should feel that way.

I'm sharing this with you, because you deserve better. We deserve better. Your child deserves better.

It may be inherently necessary that a book like this has to come with all kinds of legally approved disclaimers, but that should not prevent it from being available.

· · · · · · · ·

Here we go. You can do this. Lots of parents have walked this road before, and although it can feel achingly lonely to walk this road as a parent, you are NOT alone. I believe in you and in your child, because I know that we humans are resilient, loving, and strong. Together, we can do this.

Preface

This book is not long. That is intentional. You need something now, something simple and to the point. I know. I have been you. I am you. We live with young people who sometimes live with suicidal thoughts, and there is a shocking absence of helpful information, *practical* information, to help with the day-to-day, right-now moments of parenting a child with suicidal thoughts.

You want ideas, practical suggestions, and best practices for walking alongside your child today, this week, this season. You do not want a book on theoretical psychology of adolescents; you want to know what to do when you get them home from the hospital tomorrow, or when lunch is over today.

I know because I have been in your shoes, wanting that guidance, those suggestions, and I couldn't find them. Because I have helped raise nieces who lived with suicidal thoughts (or suicidal ideation as it is technically called), and I also have a child of my own who has lived for years with suicidal thoughts. I know the feeling of wishing someone would just hand me a simple guide with the best available information on exactly how to do this.

Because THIS is impossible. It is scary, and confusing, and there were exactly zero chapters in any of the books I read about "what to expect when you're having a baby" on how to help a child who sometimes wants to die. There is no module in the ever-popular Love & Logic parenting training on strategies for a teen who doesn't want to be alive, or just wants to be free of an emotional pain I've honestly never felt and cannot imagine.

You are leaving the immediate supervision of the standard, basic experts, but it's okay. You've done this before. No matter how thoroughly you prepared to parent your child—books you read, courses you took, research you did—there were surprises. At some point you realized that your child didn't fit the examples, or the suggested strategies didn't work for your family, and that, really, it's not even possible to adequately prepare ahead of time to be a parent. Now, you're on a whole other level, learning you can't prepare to parent a suicidal child, because there isn't a book for that.

Let's be real, you wouldn't have read that book if it had been available. Of course not! Ugh, depressing, unnecessarily alarmist. No one would buy and read that book. Not until they need it. And here you are.

Let's get the hardest part out of the way, right up front. You cannot be next to your child all day every day for the rest of their lives, or even for the next few weeks. You have to go to work, they have to go to school, you have other children, you have aging parents, you need to go grocery shopping, or you just have to go to the bathroom.

The point is that there will be a moment, a day, a week, and then a month that is not the highest point of the crisis you may be in right now, or were in last week, or whenever you've been in it. There will be a time where the 24/7 watch is over, and you and your child must head back into the rhythms of daily life.

This is *good* because it will mean your child feels like they are doing better, and you will feel they are doing better, and the expert doctors and therapists will feel they are doing better, and there is hope again.

BUT.

There is a BUT. I truly wish there wasn't, but there is.

No matter how much you love your child, how much help you get them, and how closely you watch them, even if you do every single thing right, the truth is *there is no guarantee that you can absolutely prevent your child from taking their life through suicide.*

Read that again. I know it's hard, but it's true.

No matter how much you love your child, how much help you get them and how closely you watch them, even if you do every single thing right, the truth is you cannot absolutely prevent them from taking their life through suicide.

The truth is you cannot absolutely prevent your child from taking their life through suicide.

You cannot absolutely prevent *anyone* from taking their life through suicide. There are no guarantees. Humans are impulsive, emotional creatures at best, and kids, by the inherent nature of their lack of maturity, are even MORE impulsive and emotional. When we are depressed, or hopeless, or experiencing psychosis, or in whatever state led us to suicidal thoughts, there are no absolute guarantees. As parents, we have a lot of power to recognize what's happening with our kids and intervene, AND we still can't know what we don't know.

I need you to sit with this difficult truth a minute. Sit with it, read it again, and breathe through it.

Keep breathing.

Want to throw this book across the room? It's okay, I don't mind. This is impossibly difficult, and when a good friend who is also a mental health expert told me what I just told you, it was just as gut-wrenching for me as it may be for you. It just about broke me.

I don't know for sure, but I'm guessing that whether you've been dealing with a child who is suicidal for a week or for years, no one has come right out and said to you what I just did. It's too hard, it's too scary, it's too harsh.

In fact, I think that particular hard truth is the reason that there is such scarce information on this topic for us as parents, guardians and caregivers. *(Or, for that matter, for spouses, grandparents, siblings, or friends. This book is for parents, but may be helpful for you even if you're not a parent.)* Suicidal ideation is a difficult situation, and no one wants to tell us what I just told you, **but that's not helpful**.

But—and this is a much better but—there is freedom here, and agency. Once you've processed the fact that you cannot absolutely guarantee that you can save your child's life, once you've accepted that, here's what I can promise you: the fear will actually ease, a little. It may be an imperceptible amount, but you will be able to take a slightly bigger breath, the pressure will lighten, and you will be more prepared to read, process, and implement the ideas in this book.

You will also be more prepared for the next moments with your child. You'll try something, you'll get through that, and then you'll make dinner or walk the dog or go to bed, and it will be the next day and you'll do it again. After days of getting through and then doing it again, you and your child will be on the way toward recovery from this episode of suicidal thoughts.

Here is a corollary truth that you have already, inherently, accepted, which is why I know that you can do this: as parents or caregivers, we have no guarantees about our loved ones on any given day, really. The moment they are born into this world, we know and must accept that there are risks over which we have no control, and there are illnesses and drunk drivers and injuries and bad guys and a world of things that could take them away from us or cause them harm at any minute, and we live with that every day.

Remember that moment when you and your new baby left the hospital for the first time? When maybe you and your partner looked at each other, shook your heads, and thought about heading right back inside where your baby would be safe with people who were experts, who KNEW how to handle babies? CLEARLY, you thought, that is where you and your baby should be, not on the freeway like you're just headed home with paper towels and a rotisserie chicken from Costco. But you did it. You buckled, checked, rechecked and triple-checked that car seat, and you took them home. You did it.

So, you can do this. You can. It may be *(and I hope it is)* the hardest thing you will ever do as a parent, and maybe the hardest thing you will ever do, period. But you can do this. Untold numbers of other parents have gone before you, including me. You are not alone, and together, we can do this.

Introduction

What you will find in this book, and how to use it

As you've probably already gathered, you will find real talk. Hard truths, written in the only way I know how, which I've been told generally comes across as a *(I would say 'delightful' but no one else says that)* combination of bossy and motivational. I'll share a bit from my own journey raising kids who live with suicidal thoughts: what happened, how we handled it, how we *(OK, I)* messed up, and how we got through it. I'll share strategies I've learned along the way, and resources that can help. I'll also take you through my own framework for supporting your suicidal child:

Stay Present
Communicate Openly
Advocate Fiercely
Take Care of Yourself

What you won't find in this book

There is no magic right answer, no correct sequence of steps, no three easy ways to stop your child from having suicidal thoughts. If there were, I PROMISE you I would include them, and then I would prepare for my vast riches to roll in. There is no magical answer. Anyone who tells you otherwise is lying.

How to use this book

However you want to, and however you can in the moment. You won't absorb everything right away, and some of it will seem like it's irrelevant, or too scary, or just plain not helpful right now. Skip around, read what you need, and come back to the rest when you can absorb it. It's okay.

Beyond the "No, Duh" basics

When you Google "what to do if my child is suicidal?" you will ALWAYS get the advice to call 911, or to take your child to the emergency room. I know, DUH! If you've been doing this for more than five minutes, you got that, that's not particularly helpful.

I mean, sometimes 911 or the ER is exactly what you need to do, especially if:

- your child has seriously hurt themselves.
- they are actively suicidal, with a plan and the means to complete it.
- they are actively having suicidal thoughts and you aren't sure if they are at risk for an attempt, and/or they aren't sure they can commit to not killing themself.

If that's your situation right now, you're probably not actually reading this book right now. But when you ARE in that situation, you're going to want to get your child out of immediate danger, including removing their access to harmful substances, objects, or weapons. You will want to stay with them and then get them help.

But calling 911 is primarily reserved for times when your child is at imminent risk of harming themselves. There is a whole lot of gray space between a child who is at imminent risk of harming themselves and needs to be admitted, and a child who is not at all suicidal. Gray space in which the child is, maybe, "not suicidal enough" to be admitted, but certainly not okay. When their daily reality includes thoughts of suicide or intense longing to just not be alive. When they were actively suicidal earlier this week or this month but they aren't right this minute . . . you think . . . as far as you know.

The gray space

This book is aimed squarely at that gray space, because in my experience, mental health providers, doctors and therapists don't offer much guidance for what to *actually do* in the gray space. Which is particularly unfortunate since *that gray space is where we live*, most of the time!

Some things are obvious, or they are when we're not stressed, scared, exhausted and overwhelmed: sometimes you will need to remove your child's access to all medications, sharp knives, razors, scissors, belts, ropes, etc.

But there are lots of decisions you'll need to make that are less obvious. Like, WHEN is it safe to return the knives to the kitchen drawer, or let your child have their razor back in their bathroom, and how will you know?

The bad news is that there are no magic answers, there are no exactly right answers to most of those decisions that you'll need to make. There just aren't. There is only the best decision you can make with the information you have at hand. But throughout this book, I'll share my experiences and the ideas and insight I've gathered from my research, from psychiatrists, social workers, therapists, and some REAL experts—other parents who have walked this road.

Note about terminology in this book

Just a heads up about some of the wording I'll be using:

Child/kid/teen/young adult: Statistically, most readers will have a teenager, but I'm mostly going to use the term *child* to be more age-inclusive. In fact, this book is for you if your child, teen, young adult or even your adult child is suicidal.

Mental health struggles/issue/disorder/illness: In my mind these are all interchangeable, but I use all of them just to cover my bases. The truth is that we still have a lot of stigma against mental illness, and terms like mental health struggles or mental health disorder sound less serious, and less scary. But if in fact your child is suicidal, you've probably accepted that your child is living with a brain-based illness, or mental illness. However, I use these terms interchangeably and mean the same thing with all of them.

Die by suicide/completed suicide: You may be unfamiliar with the terms "completed suicide" or "died by suicide," or they may feel awkward. You might be used to saying a person committed suicide, but think about it, what else do people commit? Adultery! Crime! Sin! Murder! But suicide is not a crime, or a moral failure. It is a function of mental illness, hopelessness, and desperation. Best practice now is to avoid the term "commit suicide" for that reason. ***Our words matter.*** One of the barriers people face sharing suicidal thoughts and asking for help is the stigma around suicide and around mental health, and some of the stigma comes from our language. It's not about being politically correct; it's about creating an environment where people feel safe being real and getting the help they need.

K, and A: K is one of my nieces, and the one for whom I've had the most responsibility as her foster parent and her aunt. A is my daughter, my middle child. Both K and A are young adults, and I share their stories with their full, informed consent, for which I am deeply grateful.

Experts: at different points in the book, I reference opinions, research, and advice from experts. Those experts, many of whom are credited in the acknowledgments, include therapists, psychologists, psychiatrists and other mental health professionals I've worked with as a caregiver, a mom, or a mental health advocate; or someone I've specifically interviewed for this book.

Why me and this book?

Who am I to write this book? Absolutely legitimate question.

Here's a quick rundown on my mental health credentials:

Spoiler alert: I am NOT a mental health provider, I am not a therapist or a doctor, so obviously I am not giving you medical advice. My perspective is one of "just" life experience. Long, hard-earned, life experience.

I do have an MBA, and I spent many years as an executive in non-profit program development. NEITHER of those experiences were the slightest bit relevant or helpful when several years ago my husband and I took in, fostered, and helped raise nieces who'd had a severely abusive childhood and were experiencing the resulting mental health issues.

I am still primary family member for those young women and have the honor to serve as legal guardian for one of them, who, in addition to her trauma and mental health issues, also lives with serious traumatic brain injury and cognitive disability.

I'm also mom to three kids, all teens or young adults. One of them lives with severe depression, ADHD, autism, and anxiety and has been hospitalized for suicidal ideation.

I am also a full-time professional mental health speaker, advocate, and mental health conference producer.

I have done a significant amount of professional training and education to better understand mental health and the experiences of people with mental illness and their families.

In the course of producing my own community mental health conferences called **Shattering Stigma with Stories**, I've spoken with hundreds of families about their experiences supporting a loved one with mental health issues.

Let me say this right off the bat. I do not claim to know your exact story, your child's exact story, and I do NOT claim to have all of the answers. No way.

In fact, maybe your experience is nothing like mine; your fears and anxieties are nothing like mine. Maybe this book will serve merely to make you feel way better about how you are handling your own experience parenting a suicidal child, and that's ok!

My family's story

When my nieces came to live with us after they had survived years of abuse by their stepfather, and they were experiencing severe mental illness as a result of that trauma, it might amuse you to know that my husband and I weren't terribly concerned. No, in fact we were quite confident! *(I always say that blissful ignorance is the best kind of ignorance.)* We thought "we're educated professionals, our parents are teachers, we've got three little boys, we've got this! We'll just love them, they'll be fine . . . we can do this."

We were WRONG.

Just two months later, I found myself sitting with a psychiatrist in an adolescent psych unit, watching my niece K on a video feed. She was only 14, she was suicidal, and she was curled in a ball on the floor of a cold bare room, terrified by uncontrollable hallucinations of her abuser. K was experiencing a life-threatening episode of mental illness.

" . . . we'll just love them; we can do this . . . "

We were SO wrong, AND wildly unprepared.

K and her sisters lived with severe complex post-traumatic stress disorder (PTSD), self-harm, depression, anxiety, and intense suicidality. The next several years were full of crises, self-harm, chaos, exhaustion, multiple suicide attempts, running away, and many long stays in the psych unit, sub-acute and residential mental health treatment. *(Side note: we were told more than once as we were preparing to take the girls in, that learning the severity of the abuse they had experienced resulted in vicarious PTSD for several of their early providers and social workers. We had no idea that was a thing, or that it would be a thing that would happen to us, but it certainly did.)*

Before my nieces lived with us, I was no different than most people. Pretty much everything I knew about mental illness, I learned in women's magazine articles. *(Those were the olden days, when people read magazines.)*

Those years as auntie, foster mom, advocate and guardian were a hard-core crash course in the difficulty and complexity of living with and treating mental illness.

We were trying to integrate the girls into school, therapy, medical appointments, and church activities. At my house that fall we had a toddler, a kindergartener, a first grader, a second grader, and a freshman in high school. The little kids were on three different soccer teams, and the teenager was in and out of the psych unit.

You know how parents will cycle through their kids' names 'til they get to the right one? I did that, and it was bad. I was calling the boys by the girls' names, the girls by the boys' names, the kids by the cats' names, the cats by the kids' names, and sometimes I was just calling out the names of random inanimate objects in desperation. "C, K, Denali, ottoman, spatula—! Would you all just put on your shoes so we can go!"

• • • • • • •

In the spirit of full disclosure, I'm just going to take a little tangent here and give you a peek into the "inherent, natural" parenting skills I brought to the table. Please note, I am an extreme extrovert. Our kids were two, five, and seven when the girls came to live with us. I had already had the oldest evaluated by early education services when he was in preschool, because I was so worried about him. I was convinced he had learning disabilities, or else something was really wrong. He rarely played with the other children at preschool, and at recess he would sit alone on the edge of the gravel area, busily stacking rocks by size, color and for all I know, geographical origin. Alone. Heartbreaking.

So, I had him evaluated, and we indeed got a diagnosis. Turns out that he had an incurable genetic condition that he would live with the rest of his life. He was, and is, an INTROVERT.

Hoo boy. This extrovert mom was a bit off base, yes?

Yeah, that's where I started. Yet overnight I was responsible for my delightful niece, who was also a self-harming and intensely suicidal teenager; and her five-year-old sister, who cried herself to sleep and during her sleep for months.

Over the next several years, I felt all of the feelings most parents, partners and family members feel at some point: terror, panic, exhaustion, helplessness, hopelessness, isolation, shame, mourning, and anger.

It's normal. When mental health problems happen to someone we know, we often don't know what to do. It can be scary or uncomfortable, and we don't want to make it worse.

Especially if:

- we don't understand the disorder.
- we feel like it's too hard, we aren't the experts, and we don't know the right things to do or say.
- we think they will always be this way and that they can't change or get better.

Can you imagine getting to a point where a suicide attempt is just one more item on a long list, no surprise, commonplace? Answering the door in the middle of night to the police, thank you ma'am, then just back to bed?

Because of the specific therapeutic treatment that K was receiving, we were instructed to NOT rush to sympathize with a suicide attempt, but instead to treat it as a behavioral choice, one that K would HAVE to get control over. *(Was that fair, given what the poor girl had been through? Nope. But it didn't matter because she was going to have to learn and practice getting to a point where suicide was no longer her go-to response for her trauma symptoms.)*

In fact, there was a night we were woken up in the wee hours of the morning by a local police officer, a knock on the door at around 2 a.m., letting us know that they had just taken K by ambulance to the hospital after another overdose attempt. As usual, we weren't even aware that she wasn't asleep downstairs in her bed. *(Alarms on doors and windows are super great, very helpful. Until the teenager figures out how to get around them.)*

Believe me, I understand, your natural response is to drop everything and rush to your child's side, rush to the hospital. It was my natural reaction as well.

Which made it all the more awkward and heartbreaking when I had to thank the lovely police officer and explain that because of her treatment, and at the direction of her psychiatrist and psychologist, we had been firmly instructed NOT to go to the hospital or even call and speak to her until the next day. *(We definitely called the hospital right away, and gave them a succinct summary of her situation, treatment and treatment team's approach.)* Similarly, because of her specific treatment for trauma and PTSD, her therapist would not speak to her for at least 24 hours if she'd either self-harmed or attempted suicide.

That night, like several other nights, we were left to just . . . go back to bed.

It was so difficult for so long. Over the years, there have been times when for my own mental health, it's felt like I've had to try and accept that despite all of the treatment, best intentions, love and care, in rare cases, suicidality might well be a terminal condition. Days when I felt so hopeless about my nieces that I had to accept that success might need to be defined as, and limited to, them knowing they were deeply loved.

This hard reality was certainly driven home many years ago in a conversation with one of K's therapists at a long-term, locked down residential facility. This therapist had come to really know and love K, in all of her goofy, kind, delightfulness. She and I were meeting to discuss

K's upcoming planned discharge back to our home, talking about how we would reintegrate her into the family after many months away, about school, and treatment, and I was feeling excited and optimistic.

The therapist stopped me and cautioned me. I needed to understand, she said, that even though K was doing well, given the level of trauma they'd been through, statistically it was highly unlikely that all four of the sisters would survive. I had to accept that even though things were better, K might still kill herself.

This is a reality those of us who are parenting suicidal kids must grapple with and accept, and I'm sure that right about now you are wondering why in the world you EVER picked up this book. *(Remember how I told you that it's OK to throw this book? Still true, although not recommended if you're reading it as an ebook on a tablet.)*

I'm sorry. I wish it wasn't true for you, or for me, or for any parent ever.

· · · · · · · ·

More recently, I experienced all of this up close and personal, when mental health challenges directly hit my nuclear family.

Our middle child had struggled with school, and with depression and anxiety, since middle school, and had been getting help for a couple of years. But we had not understood the depth of her depression, nor had we known that she had experienced hopelessness and suicidal thoughts for years. Early one morning in January of 2021, when she was 17, A came to us and told us she was very suicidal and needed to go to the hospital. We took her to the ER; A was rapidly admitted, and she spent two weeks getting intensive inpatient treatment for suicidal ideation, anxiety, depression, and previously undiagnosed ADHD *(which will be an ongoing source of mom guilt). (More mom guilt—we've since learned she is also on the autism spectrum.)*

When A went to the hospital that first time, we started at our city's best pediatric emergency room. *(This I already knew, because of my extensive history of ER visits with K.)* But they didn't have psychiatric inpatient treatment available, and so it was determined that when an adolescent bed opened up at the nearby psychiatric hospital, she would transfer there for inpatient treatment.

As is not uncommon, she had to wait more than 24 hours until that bed opened up. *(Sometimes, people have to wait several DAYS for a bed to open up if one even does, so be prepared to wait, and to possibly wait in less-than-ideal conditions.)* She was admitted to a regular hospital room to wait for the psychiatric bed, and assigned a 24-hour sitter.

If you're not familiar with the sitter situation, that is weird and uncomfortable in itself. If it is determined necessary, someone will be sitting in eyesight of your child 24 hours a day, and may even be required to be in eyesight when they use the restroom. Obviously, this can be awkward and embarrassing for the patient, even humiliating. But it is to keep them safe. *(People who are intently suicidal can be very creative about ways to hurt themselves.) (OK, it is also to protect the hospital from liability. It is what it is.)*

When it came time to transfer A, I assumed that I would pack her up and drive her to the psychiatric hospital. But I was informed that she would have to be transferred by secure medical transport.

What did that mean? It meant that a big, armed, security guard/police officer-type person escorted her in a wheelchair to a vehicle with doors that were locked from the outside, so she could not bolt. Though I asked, it was not possible for me to drive her across town myself. *(Again, liability and safety.)*

Watching my child go with an armed escort as if she was a criminal, and not a desperately ill teenager, was perhaps one of the lowest moments in this journey for me. I felt utterly hopeless, heartbroken for her, and scared. I had no idea this would be happening, so I wasn't able to prepare her. Her white-as-a-sheet, scared-but-brave face shattered me.

It was awful.

Since then, it has been a long journey trying to find adequate treatments, the right team of providers, and the right approach for the depression that will hopefully make it possible for A to fully be the loving, creative, happy person that she is meant to be.

Unfortunately, I realized that everything I'd learned about teens and suicide, before we ever knew our middle child would struggle with suicidal ideation, I'd learned directly in response to my niece K's specific situation of trauma and PTSD. Some of those lessons *(don't panic on the outside, don't freak out on the outside, how to navigate a hospital emergency room, don't forget the cell phone charger)* were appropriate and helpful.

But I realized many of those lessons, which had sunk in DEEPLY because of the traumatic situations in which I'd learned them, weren't necessarily directly transferable to our child's situation. In fact, sometimes those lessons were harmful.

Just like all of parenting, it turns out that every child and every child's situation is unique, and requires something different from us. Dang it.

· · · · · · ·

Again, I have both K and A's full permission to share. I've been sharing K's story with her permission for years, and, in fact, when I asked A, she said, *(let's be honest, while rolling her eyes)* "Of course, Mom, I'm not HIDING anything." Our kids often have a far healthier attitude about mental health problems than we do.

Note: I hope you've picked up that I write about K and A in the present tense, and there is a brief update on each of them at the end of this book. But whether you skip ahead to that or not, know that recovery may be hard work, but it is real and it is possible.

First things first

Wait, what is even happening?

If your child has never had mental health problems before now, or if they've struggled but they've never been suicidal before, here's a quick, mini crash course: First, take a deep breath. I don't mean that in a patronizing or scolding way. But when your child is suicidal, you aren't thinking or processing at your best because you are scared. Taking a deep breath will help calm your overactivated nervous system and regulate your breathing, your heartbeat, and your thinking.

Anytime you start to feel like you are breathing shallowly, feeling extra anxious, or your thoughts start racing with worry, STOP. Breathe. Even three deep breaths in and out will make a difference, telling your nervous system that you're okay and you're in control.

You know now that your child needs help, though you may not know, yet, what that help should look like. This is GOOD news, honest. There are SO many approaches and strategies to help your child, and to help you help your child on their journey toward healing and wholeness.

People imagine that the state of being suicidal is a singular moment. Get through the moment, and you'll be okay. Unfortunately, it's usually not like that. First, by the time you know someone else is suicidal, they've likely felt that way a long time. And they will likely continue to feel that way for some amount of time.

Believe it or not, suicidal thoughts are a common and even normal part of the human experience. It happens to many, many people, which may surprise you if it hasn't happened to you. It's important to remember that having suicidal thoughts doesn't mean someone will attempt suicide, nor does it mean dying by suicide is inevitable. Suicidal thoughts aren't pleasant, and they aren't comfortable, but those thoughts don't have to translate to dying by suicide. **Suicidal thoughts don't have to translate to dying by suicide.**

In fact, most people who have suicidal thoughts will not attempt suicide, and most who attempt suicide will not die by suicide. Some studies have found that 90% of people who attempt suicide will go on to die of something other than suicide.

Sometimes suicide is an impulsive response to overwhelming hopelessness and emotional pain; sometimes it is a poor coping strategy; sometimes it is a chosen behavior. In the long term, treatment strategies and therapeutic strategies may be different, but in the short-term immediate moment, the steps are the same: Keep your child physically safe, get them rest and good nutrition, help them get re-centered, keep them surrounded, if possible, by their safe people, and distract them.

Getting your child help

If your child is struggling with suicidal thoughts, it is clear you need to get them help. As I've said, what may not be clear is exactly what that means or how to access it. It's okay to just start. You don't have to know exactly what help your child needs, you just need to start talking to people, getting advice, and asking questions. If it's not an immediate, life-threatening emergency, I would recommend that you start with their pediatrician or primary care provider, who can ask you questions, talk to your child, and then recommend and connect you with resources and next steps.

Getting your child help with suicidal thinking can mean connecting them with a psychiatrist for an evaluation and possible medical treatment, or finding a therapist for ongoing support. There are also many other levels and types of care, including subacute care, residential treatment; intensive outpatient, partial hospitalization, or day treatment programs; or inpatient hospitalization. All of these options will depend on your child's needs, what your insurance will cover/what you can pay for, and what programs have openings at that time.

Most important? Just start. Pick up the phone.

Beyond 911: 988

One of the first things I want you to know, if you are in the United States, is the National Suicide & Crisis Lifeline: 988 (988lifeline.org). You or your child can call, text, or chat online with a trained crisis counselor who can listen, be present, and provide guidance on the most appropriate next steps and resources. This lifeline is available 24/7. In their own words, 988 counselors "will listen to you, understand how your problem is affecting you, provide support, and share resources that may be helpful."

I want you to understand 988 and be ready to use it, and make sure your child and your other family members have it in their phone.

Seriously, get your phone out. I'll wait. Open up a new contact and add 988. I know you're thinking "seriously, Tara, it's three numbers, I'll remember." But in a crisis our brains and our memory sometimes fail us, and how great to know it's in there already.

You and your child should know that calling 988, or any crisis line, is not like going to McDonald's. It will not be the exact same experience every time; it will not always be equally helpful; and not every counselor you connect with will have the same personality, approach, skills or training. I've definitely had people tell me that it wasn't helpful, that they felt that the information provided was very basic and scripted, and they weren't provided additional resources.

HOWEVER, many lives have been saved by the fantastic people (mental health professionals or trained volunteers) who staff the crisis lines, and each experience depends on who answers the phone. I have a friend who lives with suicidal thinking and has needed to call a crisis line for herself on more than one occasion. When she calls the crisis line, and she is not "vibing" with the first person on the other end of the line, if they aren't helpful, or she doesn't feel heard, she politely hangs up (politely, because she is delightful even when suicidal), waits a minute, and calls back to reach someone else. It's okay.

Calling 988 is appropriate when you need emergency help and there is no immediate physical threat of danger—no weapons, no physical injury, no violence is involved. If that is NOT the case, and the situation is dangerous or someone needs immediate medical attention, you should call 911.

If you do call 911, be very clear with the dispatcher and with any first responders that your child is having a mental health crisis, and you would like them to send crisis intervention trained (CIT) officers, who have special training in mental health issues and ways to help.

When should you go to the ER?

If your child is talking about suicide, if they have a plan for how they might attempt suicide, if you are concerned they will attempt suicide, or if you are concerned about their physical safety or the risk they might hurt anyone else, you should absolutely go to the emergency room.

Other reasons to consider taking your child to the emergency room for mental health concerns include if they are experiencing:

- visual or auditory hallucinations
- delusions
- severe medication side effects
- severe insomnia
- aggression or assault
- paranoia
- confusion
- mania

A sad reality about our current broken mental health system is often the best or only path to accessing higher-level care for your child runs through the emergency room. *I am referring to the mental health system in the U.S., as that is where I live and what I know. Health system specific advice may not be applicable if you live somewhere else, but much of the rest of the book will apply no matter where you or your child are.*

As unfortunate, inefficient, and suboptimal as the path is, that's the path our mental health system takes. You may need to keep that in mind even if you aren't sure that your child's life is immediately at risk. It is possible that as you search for help, you may reach a dead-end which will require a trip to the emergency room to make any progress in securing additional help or resources for your child.

Taking them to the emergency room

If you have had any time to prepare for this possibility, you have time to do some research. If you haven't had time to plan, you need to do that research now, quickly. Is there a pediatric hospital in your community? Do they have inpatient psychiatric care, in case it's needed, and do they have a psychiatric focus in their emergency department? Which hospital is in your insurance plan? Do any of those hospitals have inpatient pediatric psychiatric units, in case your child needs to be admitted?

What does and doesn't happen at the ER

The first time I took K to the emergency room because she was suicidal, and she was admitted to the adolescent psychiatric unit, I was so relieved. *Ok,* I thought, *that was scary but now we're getting somewhere, now we'll get this figured out and fixed!*

My ~~innocence~~ shocking naiveté back then was adorable.

First, I learned that the term *psychiatric evaluation* does not really mean what I thought it meant, at least not at the ER or even in a hospital psych unit. A full psychiatric evaluation will be done when you're NOT in crisis, and will be an appointment or a series of appointments that take place over several hours. This type of evaluation is thorough, delves into your child's entire medical and developmental history, and can help parse out exactly what is going on with your child, including whether or not there is more than one issue involved (known as co-occurring disorders or co-morbidities.)

But a psych evaluation in the ER is MUCH more limited. Really, the purpose of an ER psych eval is to answer three questions:

1. Medical clearance: Is this truly a psychiatric event, or is there possibly another medical explanation for what is happening? (Think substance use, accidental poisonings, infections that can cause hallucinations, a brain tumor, carbon monoxide poisoning, etc.) One of the first things that may happen is that your child will get drug and other toxicology testing.

2. If it is a psychiatric event, are they an immediate danger of harm to themselves?

3. If it is a psychiatric event, are they an immediate danger of harm to others?

Whether or not your child is admitted to the hospital will depend on, among other things, if the medical professionals conclude the answer to either of the last two questions is yes.

At the ER, a social worker or psychologist will interview your child, and then you, often separately, as well as with the two of you together. Be prepared that the medical personnel might not tell you everything your child has said. That's part of the process, and the most important thing is that your child tells SOMEONE the truth about what they are experiencing. Don't be upset or offended by this. The truth is that sometimes kids will be more honest with strangers than they will with us, and that's especially true with information they fear will get them in trouble or upset us or make us sad. The most important thing right now is that the medical professionals get the most complete, accurate picture of what your child is struggling with.

When you are talking to the doctors or social workers, be certain, clear, and concise about your concerns for their safety. DO NOT

MINIMIZE anything. It is tempting as a parent to avoid appearing like we are exaggerating or being dramatic, and we want to make our family members look good. We may not even do it consciously. Or maybe we don't want to potentially be judged as bad parents by the medical professionals. But this is not the time to be understated. To get your child the help they need, you need to be fully honest with the medical professionals. Be ready to share exactly what made you concerned enough to bring your child into the ER, what they said, what plans they may have shared, or actions they have taken that indicate they are serious about suicide.

Keeping a history of your child's symptoms, medications, treatments such as therapy, and behaviors is important because in the ER is not the time to give doctors a long, drawn-out story about your child's entire life, that one thing they did that one time a few years ago, what they were like in preschool, etc. Medical personnel don't have time for that, frankly. If you aren't direct and clear about your immediate concerns for safety and the severity of the situation, they may get impatient, and your child may not get the attention or treatment they need. Real talk.

I'm repeating myself but it's important. You're going to be tempted to leave out the worst bits, the bits that make your child seem like a bad kid, or might make you seem like a bad parent, or that might make your child seem really ill. DON'T. If your child has been using cannabis/marijuana, or drinking alcohol, or using other substances, tell them. The ER staff can't give your child the help they need if you aren't fully forthcoming. They **won't** give your child the help they need if you aren't fully forthcoming. Tell them everything, and *(to the extent possible)* be ready to tell them CONCISELY.

Sometimes, just the act of going to the emergency room, sitting long enough to get really bored, and talking through what they are feeling will be enough to help your child regulate. There were a few times we took K to the ER and were sent home that same day, sometimes simply because after a few long hours of waiting around, she said she no longer planned to kill herself . . . that day.

Turns out, it is possible to be suicidal but not quite suicidal enough. And honestly, even though it is scary for you, suicidal thinking can sometimes be appropriately managed from home with your child's team. Hospitalization is used when a person can't or hasn't kept themselves safe.

Also . . .

Ugh.

Let's just stop right here and acknowledge the vast gulf in comfort levels between an ER psychiatric professional and a parent with the conclusion "well, we're pretty sure they won't kill themselves tonight, so we don't need to admit them." Especially if the answer to "But how do you KNOW for sure?" is "because they told us so."

What I learned is that hospital psychiatric stays are purely for stabilization for people who aren't safe in the moment, safe to themselves or to others. It is NOT for comprehensive treatment. Stays are measured in days, usually, or a couple of weeks, and revolve around getting your child stabilized.

WHAT TO BRING TO THE ER FOR A PSYCH EVALUATION

☐ Full list of all current medications

☐ History of all medications used in the past

☐ If an overdose is suspected, bring whatever medication or substance you think they took.

☐ Ready description of what your child is like when they are well

☐ Contrasting, specific and non-minimizing description of current symptoms and behaviors

☐ Phone charger and extra power source if possible

☐ An expectation that you will be there for several hours, so:

- Get someone else to pick up the kids.
- Get someone else to feed the dogs.
- Tell work you are out for the day (and probably tomorrow).

☐ Insurance information and ID

☐ Cash for the vending machines

☐ A water bottle

☐ Phone numbers and contact info for your child's current doctors

☐ Book, tablet, headphones *(I know, you think that you'll never be able to focus on anything else in these circumstances. But no matter how dramatic or traumatic the event that brought you in, once your child is safe in the immediate moment, the adrenaline will fade. After a while you will both get bored, and the* People *magazine from 1998 won't cut it. Take my word for it.)*

☐ You should both wear comfortable clothes, if possible, you'll likely be sitting for a while. And layers. And maybe a blanket. You will be either too hot or too cold, more likely too cold.

If your child is admitted to the hospital

If you suspect *(or hope! That's ok.)* that your child will be admitted, bring them an overnight bag with:

- Comfortable clothes without a drawstring *(unlikely to be allowed in the psych unit)*
- Slip on shoes without laces *(also not usually allowed)*
- Bras with no underwire *(also not usually allowed)*
- A small comfort item such as a favorite stuffy, pillow, or blanket from home.

If your child is admitted, make sure not to leave them with:

- Any valuables, including jewelry, expensive electronics, phones, etc. *(Phones may or may not be allowed. If allowed, and you decide to leave the phone, know there is a chance it may disappear.)*

Every facility has different rules, of course, and some items from home may not be allowed. Also be aware that it is likely that everything you bring into the hospital will be taken from you first by staff, thoroughly searched for safety, and then catalogued before being given back to your child. Keep in mind that even if you are one hundred percent certain an item would be safe for your child, it might not be safe for another child, and staff are responsible for keeping all of the kids on the unit safe. *(Even then, a person determined to harm themselves can be incredibly clever at finding ways to do that. So, when inpatient staff refuse to let your child have a pair of fingernail clippers, don't get annoyed or offended, trust them. And when they insist on searching the socks you packed yourself, and they find a cigarette lighter you missed and confiscate it, thank them! Because a really determined suicidal teenager can do some serious damage to themselves with just about anything.) (Why yes, that was an oddly specific personal example . . . sigh.)*

While in the hospital your child may see a therapist at least once a day; a psychiatrist once or more during their stay; they will also likely have group therapy each day, maybe more than once; and some quiet time that might include crafts or school-like worksheets. The environment is hopefully quiet and restful, though it is structured, with set mealtimes and group times.

If it is a weekend, they may not see a therapist or a psychiatrist, as weekends are much quieter with fewer "treatment" activities.

Communicating with your child during their stay

While your child is in the hospital, you will probably be allowed to visit at certain times, generally when there are no therapy groups or other important activities happening. You can also speak to them on the phone, though that might be a brief and frustrating exercise since it's often a shared, public phone. Each facility will have their own rules: when they can talk to you on the phone; when you can visit; what you can bring; and where they can go with you during a visit (likely not away from the facility).

Even if visits and phone calls are brief or inconvenient, they are important for your child, and you need to make reasonable efforts to make it happen. This will reassure your child that you aren't angry at them, or disappointed in them, and that you still love them. *(Of course you do, but your child isn't doing their best thinking at the moment. They need your reassurance.)* Now, it is also entirely possible, especially if your child is a teen, that they may not always be in the mood to talk, and they may either be very brief or may actually refuse a visit or phone call. As painful as that is for you, keep trying. They are going through a life-threatening mental health episode, and it's a lot. But the act of you trying reminds them they are loved, even if they aren't feeling lovable or they are angry or confused.

You can also call the nurses' station or staff to request an update on how your child is doing. I often called in the late evening, before I went to bed, so I could get some assurance that my child was safe and settled for the night. *(Just remember that hospitals and facilities are often understaffed, so be concise and reasonable in the amount of time and attention you are requesting.)*

Visits

Outside of family therapy sessions and professionally guided conversations, it's best to keep visits light. Visits don't need to be long; 15-20 minutes can be enough to check in, remind your child you are there for them, and that you love them. Be supportive of the process and validate your child's fears or frustrations, AND also validate their effort. Tell them how proud you are of the work they are doing.

Ask the staff first, of course, but you can often bring snacks or treats from outside, to break up the routine of hospital food. Your child may also need or want you to bring clean clothes, different comfort items from home *(as long as they are allowed)*, or things they can work on during quiet times. Bring books, or colored pens for journaling, or a favorite blanket or comfort item, IF ALLOWED.

Because I was often visiting my niece with my three young children, we would bring crafts or a game to play, and we would frequently show up with a milkshake and French fries.

There is something difficult or even surreal about drinking a chocolate shake while having awkward conversations with your child about their siblings, their pets or the activities at home, all while knowing full well that your child is very depressed and in fact wants to die. It's okay, it IS awkward, at best.

But remember, much of recovery is minute by minute, getting through one thing and then another, until you and your child are building resilience and remembering "normal" simply by getting through to the next moment. It's okay to play UNO or eat fries together. In fact, that can be one underappreciated blessing of a hospitalization or other residential stay.

You have likely been under a tremendous amount of stress, possibly watching your child like a hawk, constantly worried about their physical safety, and exhausted from it all. Now, you can just relax a bit, and remind your child and yourself of a different, healthier dynamic that is available to you while they are safe: a dynamic that is not based on fear and anticipation and vigilance, but simply based on enjoying your child, being present with them, and letting them know they are loved.

Trust the process, and help your child trust the process

Finally, realize that no matter your child's age, but especially if they are a teen, this is their time and their healing journey. This may be the first time that you have had to fully relinquish your perceived control of your child, but your child has work to do, work that you cannot do for them. You cannot control this, you cannot fix this, you cannot do this for them, and you have to yield them to the experts *(while doing all of the due diligence, supervision and participation possible.)* I know, this is impossibly difficult, especially when you may be used to being extremely involved in managing their days and their moods and their behaviors and . . .

Truthfully, mental illness is one of the only medical conditions I can think of in which the person experiencing the problem is responsible for doing so much of the work to get better. While medications are likely to be an important part of your child's healing journey, they are not a magic bullet, and the rest of the healing is your child's work to do.

Your child may be angry they are in the hospital, they may be relieved that they are safe, they may be discouraged and more depressed. They might lash out at you in anger with unkind words, or they may not feel like visiting. It's not about you, it's about them, and what they are going through is just as scary for them as it is for you. Be compassionate. Let them know you wish this wasn't necessary, but you are proud of them. Assure them that their feelings are okay, that you can handle their feelings, and that they are going to feel better, eventually.

What you should do while your child is hospitalized

Go home— Really. I know, it's brutal. I have made that hard, hard walk out of the hospital into the parking lot without my child. It felt wrong on every level. As parents or guardians, we are used to taking care of our kids ourselves. WE kiss the boo-boos, WE bandage the scrapes, WE hug them when they are sad.

They have to walk out their own journey now. It feels against the natural order, but this is something they can only do for themselves, with the help of those specially trained to walk this journey with them.

We can't do it for them, and it's so freaking hard. But it is also the thing they need, and that will make them stronger. They are receiving the medical care they need and the coping skills they need to begin healing, and that healing will bring them strength and wholeness. What you could provide at home was not enough, and they need more. You are not abandoning them, although it may feel that way as you sit alone in the car in the parking lot after each visit. You are helping them in the best way you can, with the best resources you can access, and you are supporting them, loving them, and cheering them on. This is parenting at its most difficult and its best.

Also, congratulations. No, really. You realized your child needed serious intervention, you successfully advocated for them, and you got them admitted to the hospital, or to a longer-term residential treatment facility. That's a huge accomplishment, even though it may be an accomplishment you never wanted.

Sleep—your child is safe, and you are exhausted: from fear, hypervigilance, crisis, and drama. This is the time to rest, recharge, and be as fresh as possible for when they come home. Make this a priority, because hospital stays can be unpredictable in length, and you don't know how long the stay will last.

Remove all dangerous items or lock them up—Get a lock box for: all medications (both over-the-counter and prescription); alcohol; knives and scissors; and anything else your child has considered using in a suicide attempt (remember, it's okay to ask them directly, and you can also talk to their providers). This isn't forever, it's just for right now. (Often hospitals, related nonprofits or other organizations have free lock boxes, so ask around. You can also purchase them.)

Make sure that when they get home, your child will not have access to credit cards or large amounts of cash, and therefore the ability to buy pills or a firearm on the internet, or from coworkers or friends. Consider friends and family that they may visit. Be ready to monitor and also have hard conversations with those folks about access to medications and firearms, to help protect your child.

Consider whether you need to lock up or hide car keys.

Check in with siblings, other family members—this is traumatic for the whole family, and while your child is hospitalized is the perfect time to check in with everyone else. Spend some extra time giving other siblings TLC, talking things out with your spouse or partner, etc.

Think about what YOU need, and ask for it—People will offer to help. At least they will once and IF you tell them what's going on. Start there. Think of a small group of friends, family members, and even coworkers or your boss with whom you can share what's going on, so they can support you.

Cancel everything you can—work, volunteer activities, other obligations. A family member in the hospital can be intense and time-demanding, and a psychiatric hospitalization is no exception. You will likely have

multiple meetings or calls with your child's treatment team, family therapy sessions, and visits with your child, and you will have to work your
schedule around the facility's schedule.

Sleep some more—Can you tell what one of my primary coping mechanisms is?

Don't be afraid to ask questions—Be sure you understand what medications your child may be receiving, and what the overall treatment
goals are during their stay. If you don't understand something, ask for
clarification. The doctors and therapists are definitely busy, but they
want to know if you are confused or if you are concerned about an
aspect of treatment.

Discharge

Understand that a psychiatric hospitalization is not about "fixing" your
child or curing them. Psychiatric hospitalization is about keeping your
child safe in an immediate emergency; stabilizing them until they are
safe to go home; and doing a holistic evaluation of your child's diagnosis and treatment plan that they can then pass off to your child's
outpatient providers, such as their psychiatrist or therapist, and their
primary care provider.

At some point, after a few days, a week, or maybe longer, the treatment team will decide that your kid is stabilized and ready to be discharged. Stabilized, not well, because remember, treatment and recovery
are not the goal of a hospital admission, just stabilization. They may
have re-evaluated or changed medications, done an initial assessment,
and they feel like your child is ready, or more realistically, safe enough
to go home.

This may be a scary time for you AND your child. After all, if they
were at imminent risk just a few days ago, how could it possibly be okay
to send them home already? That is a natural concern, and it's normal
to be worried.

ITEMS TO LOCK UP WHILE YOUR LOVED ONE IS SUICIDAL

This list may be different for you and your loved one. Think about what they have planned or thought about using to harm themselves. Talk to them about what items are unsafe for them, and consult with their providers for more information. Also, see resources in the appendix from the Treatment Advocacy Center for a more thorough discussion.

- ☐ All medications: prescription, over the counter and recreational/illegal

- ☐ Alcoholic beverages

- ☐ Toxic cleaning substances

- ☐ Knives, scissors and other sharps

- ☐ All guns and ammunition

- ☐ Cords, ties, ropes, etc.

- ☐ Credit cards (to prevent purchase of drugs or weapons)

- ☐ Car keys

When the team is talking about discharge, it is important that the next steps are clear.

- Does your child have follow-up appointments set with a psychiatrist or psychiatric nurse practitioner, and/or their therapist, as appropriate? In an ideal world, you should have these appointments before you leave the hospital. We do not live in an ideal world, and provider and resource shortages may make it impossible. But TRY, and if you can't get them lined up, know you will have to push for them ASAP, and keep calling.

- Do you have prescriptions for all of their medications? Do you both know when a return to the emergency room would be necessary?

- Finally, do you have a thorough safety plan?

You may notice in your treatment planning, whether on discharge from a facility or other times in the journey, a focus on what your child needs to feel safe right now. In my conversations with experts for this book, it seems there has been a shift from a focus on risk assessment—with a focus on suicidal thoughts, plans, access to items of harm, set time/day—to a focus on what is needed right now? What can create safety for the person now and in the future?

The experts with whom I spoke believe that in many ways a risk assessment focus is fear based, and the second approach—on creating safety in the here and now—is a more effective approach that brings hope, builds bridges, and builds capacity in the individual and in the relationship.

Treatment planning

You should not be discharged without a plan for next steps. Your child may be stabilized from the recent crisis, but the underlying issues that caused the crisis, and caused their suicidal ideation, are still there.

To that end, what does the hospital or facility think are your child's underlying issues? This is a critical piece of information to get before you bring your child home, because it will differentiate the path in front of you:

- If you know what the underlying issues are, then you know that you need a treatment team with expertise in those issues.

- If you don't know what the underlying issues are, then that means you need more information. You need a better assessment and/or a deeper psychiatric evaluation before you can build a good treatment plan.

Sometimes your child will be discharged home and connected with therapy and/or a psychiatrist for ongoing support. Sometimes the hospital may recommend other levels of care, including subacute care or residential treatment (both types of care at facilities where your child lives onsite for weeks or months). Alternatively, they may recommend that your child goes home and participates in an intensive outpatient, partial hospitalization, or day treatment program, in which they sleep at home but spend a varying number of days each week traveling to a place where they can get ongoing group therapy, skills training, and other more intensive therapeutic services. All of these options will depend on what your child's needs are, what your insurance will cover/what you can pay for, and what programs have openings at that time. The team at the hospital, your child's own psychiatrist or therapist, and perhaps an insurance company case manager should all work together to help you make the best plan for next steps.

As their parent or caregiver, you have the right to challenge a discharge plan and push for one that is more thorough, better addresses your specific concerns, or connects you with more robust resources for your child. Be clear about your concerns and ask questions.

Safety planning

A safety plan is a document that your child will draft with the help of their providers and with you, and that will be agreed on by the team. This is the place where the team will decide if medications and sharps need to be locked up, and if there are other dangerous items in the home that should be removed. It is also the place where your child will make a plan for what they will do if they feel suicidal—Who will they call? Where will they go? What are the steps they can take to stay out of crisis? What will you do?

You, your child, and their provider *(therapist, psychiatrist, psych nurse practitioner, etc.)* will come up with this plan, and you'll each agree to it. Ideally your child should be actively involved, since the point of the plan is to list things they can do when they are struggling. A standardized plan with suggestions of what to do in a crisis might be offered, but your child is less likely to use it or feel it's helpful if it isn't individualized for them. The team should try and help your child think about what they know can help and what makes things worse for them when they are in a crisis. As the parent or caregiver, you should be given the opportunity to review and provide input, and you should also have a copy so you can help support them in following their safety plan.

Since it is not super practical to carry around a paper plan, you should know there are several free safety plan apps available that can be downloaded to use on your child's phone, such as SafetyPlan, Suicide Safety Plan, and Virtual Hope Box.

The safety plan also needs to be shared with your child's school and with their primary care provider. Your child's school may require a safety plan for them to return, and schools and hospitals can and should share a safety plan back and forth with your permission.

Safety plans should be developed for each of your child's environments, as resources and triggers will differ from home to school, or from one parent's home to another. So, you will need different plans for each of those environments, taking into account which trusted adults would be available in each environment; what your child can do to distract themselves during difficult moments when at home or at school; and what other steps need to be taken for them to feel safe.

· · · · · · · ·

Then *(and this is where it gets hard for a scared parent, not going to lie to you)*, based simply on the word of the child who is struggling with suicidal thoughts, they will send you and your child home. Right now, reading this book in the privacy of wherever you are reading this book, is the appropriate time and place to scream with your outside *(or inside, if you have to)* voice, "Are you freaking kidding me? This is the best practice??? You are sending my child home simply based on their word that they are no longer suicidal, and on their word that they will follow this safety plan??? Just in the last week they lied to me about their homework, the laundry, and whether they ate the last Oreo! The stakes are a good bit higher right now!"

Well, yes, unfortunately. What are the options? Keeping your child locked up forever? Generally frowned upon, even in this situation. At some point, your child must agree to stay alive, and you must give them the trust and dignity of respecting that, even when maybe you are both scared it won't really stay true.

Discharge? Already?

You may be tempted to stall discharge. I get it, and I've been there. You may not feel ready, you may not feel your child is ready, and you are scared. Certainly, you can and should share your concerns as specifically and logically and factually as you can with the treatment team. Your perspective on your child is important, and if you truly believe that it is too soon for discharge, you should let them know.

However, the realities of our mental health care system are that there aren't enough beds, insurance won't cover as much as we often think they should, and at some point, your child needs to transition to the next stage of their healing.

You will need to summon your strength, manage your fear, and make sure the message that your child receives is NOT "this is terrifying, I don't think you can do this, this is a disaster." Instead, the message they need to get from you and their team is "we know this is hard, you've been through a lot, but you are strong, we are here with you, and you are going to be ok."

DON'T LEAVE THE HOSPITAL WITHOUT:

☐ A specific number (ideally an on-call cell number) at the hospital you can call to reach a social worker, a nurse or other provider if you have problems in the first few days at home

☐ A thorough plan—including next appointments set with appropriate mental health providers—for follow-up care that you feel good about, and that you feel like you can sustain.

☐ A safety plan that you and your child have both agreed to.

☐ Specific advice on what to do if your child has suicidal thoughts or plans. Know what to look for that would indicate you need to consider bringing your child back to the hospital.

☐ A to-do list of appointments to make, medications to fill, etc.

☐ A thorough understanding of your child's medication regimen, especially if it has been changed.

☐ Removing or locking up all medications, weapons, sharps and other items of concern at home as indicated by conversations with your child and the providers.

☐ Any electronics (tablets, game devices, cell phones) if they were allowed, and all chargers. *(I mean, the last thing you need right now is a charger crisis!)*

Coming home from a hospitalization

Bringing your child home from a psychiatric hospitalization is a lot—a lot of emotions, expectations, and fears.

You are so happy they are home. It was weird for them to be gone, and your family unit felt off. Plus, them coming home from the hospital means that healing and recovery has begun. Plus, there's a little voice deep inside that hopes that maybe things will go back to normal now.

Here's the deal. Things won't go back to normal, but you will find a new normal.

There are helpful aspects of a hospital stay that you can replicate at home, especially in those first few days after they come home. In the first few days, everyone is likely to be relieved and then nervous. Focus on creating a calm, safe environment.

The first thing to remember is that your child is recovering from a bout of mental illness, and that recovery requires some of the same things required when recovering from physical injury or illness. Remember, brain health is physical health. Mental health crises are physical health crises. Therefore, your child has just experienced a serious health crisis. They need what anyone needs after a serious health crisis. *(So do you, so don't skip the section later in the book on taking care of yourself.) (No, seriously, don't.)*

What would you do if you had just brought your child home from the hospital after surgery? Those are basically the things your child needs right now. The basics, like lots of rest, extra TLC, reduced expectations at school and in life, comforting foods, and probably Netflix or YouTube.

They need rest, quiet, distraction from discomfort, extra attention, comforting nutrition, and sleep. Chicken noodle soup, crackers, and a 7-Up *(or was that just my childhood comfort food on a sick day?)* are never a bad thing, whether you have the flu or a mental health crisis.

Someone who has experienced a major suicidal depression can take a year or even longer to fully recover. Think of it like this: in a way, your child has had a "brain attack." In that time, they need much of what someone recovering from major surgery or a heart attack or stroke would need: rest, good nutrition, support from their community, rest, adjusted expectations, and extra medical attention.

You will have follow-up appointments to schedule and attend with either regular providers such as psychiatrists and therapists, or with new providers. There may be new medications to fill and new conversations to schedule with the school team. A to-do list will be your friend right now, as your brain and spirit are also still recovering from the trauma of your child's illness and hospitalization, and you likely aren't operating at peak performance levels.

Managing expectations for everyone is key to a successful re-entry. There will be bumps in the road. It's important to remember your child isn't cured, they aren't all better—they were merely (hopefully) stabilized. Their depression, anxiety or other underlying issues aren't gone, but the hope is that for right now, those issues are less intense and overwhelming.

You're scared, but remember your child is also probably scared, nervous about the possibility of a return of intense suicidality. The first few hours or days home can be kind of a honeymoon, with everyone just relieved and happy that your child is home. This is a perfect time to begin talking *(or re-emphasize if it was discussed during family therapy before they left the hospital)* about the fact that there will be bumps, that they are to be expected and even planned for. Talk about how your child might communicate difficult feelings to you more quickly; how they can tell things might be headed in the wrong direction; how you might be able to tell things might be headed in the wrong direction; and you can discuss and agree on ways you can be helpful. This also allows your child to tell you what you might do that is UNHELPFUL, and perhaps what you might do that actually drives them crazy, and you can, within reason, reshape your responses accordingly. *(I found out early on from my niece that following her around asking "Are you suicidal now? How about now? Are you thinking of killing yourself now?" was really not helpful to her. Go figure.)*

Helpful things about the hospital you can replicate

Routine: This is the time to focus on regular bedtimes and mealtimes. Days in the hospital were likely quite regimented around mealtime, therapy, group therapy, craft time, etc.

While they may have chafed at all of that structure, it also can be a relief for many kids whose days are normally either heavily scheduled and/or chaotic, reducing anxiety and uncertainty. Maintaining some of that quiet, routine and structure at home may be helpful as your child re-enters their "normal" life, in terms of regular sleep schedules, some minimal expectations for chores or homework, and intentional connection with family and friends.

School: If they can work on schoolwork, or when they are up to going to school (and everyone involved deems that safe and appropriate), great, especially if it's a positive distraction, but this isn't the time to stress out about school either. Life has taken a turn, and school will be there when they're ready. *(You may need to reread that last sentence several times. Go ahead. School can be a particularly hard piece for parents to release, but for now your child is on a different journey. It's okay. School will be there when they're ready.)*

You can also encourage them to continue with any new activities that they may have found helpful in the hospital, such as journaling or crafting. *(But be ready for them to reject that suggestion, as my child did, right after I bought the largest available set of gel markers and some adult coloring books. Not THAT kind of adult coloring books, more like pretty flowers and stuff. Oh, well. Maybe I'll use them to reduce MY anxiety.)*

Your presence: They may be grateful for the restoration of privacy, their own bed, blanket and belongings, but coming home to hours and hours alone in their room is an abrupt adjustment. It's not a great idea to leave them entirely to their own devices, even if they say they just want to be left alone.

You will want to keep a close eye on your child when they come home *(and any time they are actively suicidal, especially if they feel unsafe.)* That may mean popping in to their room regularly with snacks; asking them to stay in eyesight of you in the living room or kitchen; having them shadow you or accompany you on errands and around the house for chores; or even having them sleep on the floor in your room or vice versa, depending on what you, your child and their team think is appropriate. Basically, the message is "Welcome to being attached at the hip." It isn't punishment—it's for their safety. This isn't forever, and it won't be anything new for a child who's been in a hospital or facility. While they were there, they had people checking on them constantly. So this won't be a new practice to them, even if it's new to you. If not, that's okay, you do it anyway.

They may think you're being weird, and they **will** think it's annoying even if they're used to it from the hospital. It's okay to come straight out and say that you need them to stay close to you or tolerate your face more frequently than normal until they are out of this current crisis.

You can ease up on this as feels most appropriate for your child or tighten up when they are having a particularly hard moment or day.

Safe environment: An adolescent psychiatric unit is a safe place. Similarly, at home, there should not be anything accessible with which your child could easily injure themselves. You need to replicate that environment in your home, whether or not they have been hospitalized. You will need to become familiar with protective measures around lethal safety measures and safe storage options. That includes locked storage for medicines (including prescriptions, OTC and vitamins/supplements); sharps (including knives, razors, broken glass, needles, etc.); and firearms. If you don't have a lockbox for medications and sharps, the hospital may be able to provide you with one, or you can order them on Amazon.

There may be other objects you need to remove from the environment, depending on what your child's thoughts or plans for suicide have included. Ask them. Again, you will not put ideas in their head. Let them help you keep them safe by asking them what they have contemplated in the past, and if there is anything in the environment that makes them feel unsafe.

If you are concerned about your child leaving their room at night, or leaving your home, you can use door chimes or alerts to help you know when that might be happening.

At the same time, if someone is extremely determined to take their life, it can be difficult to think of everything. Hopefully because your child was released, they are not at immediate elevated risk, but risk levels can change. Healing is not a linear process, and rehospitalization or residential treatment is sometimes necessary and appropriate. If you need to return to the ER to have your child evaluated because you don't think you can keep them safe, you can, don't hesitate.

A Note on Guns

If you have a child who has experienced suicidal ideation, it is my deeply held opinion that you should not have **any** firearms in the home. None. It simply isn't worth the risk. Teens and children are impulsive, and people who are suicidal can be impulsive, and firearms make it all too easy to act on an impulse. Store them off-site, locked up, with a friend or relative, and don't tell your child where they are.

I am not anti-gun, I'm anti-regret. *(Honest. No agenda here, just reality. I grew up in a family of hunters, and truly am not anti-gun. But it's NOT safe for a person who is suicidal to have ANY access to firearms. Period.)*

If the gun(s) MUST be in your home, they must be locked in a gun cabinet, with a password that is NOT accessible to your child, away from any ammunition, in a way that takes time to access. Please. This is not a regret that you want to live with.

Risk of post-discharge time period

It is also important to acknowledge that for some kids, discharge and the period of time at home immediately after a psychiatric inpatient stay can actually be a time of increased risk. Although the immediate crisis has passed, the underlying issues that caused your child to struggle in the first place are certainly still there. In fact, with the immediate crisis resolved and the fog of a suicidal episode disbursed, space opens up for your child to begin really thinking about and engaging with those underlying issues. This is good, because it means the real work of healing is beginning, and it is hard, because healing can be difficult, and the process can result in the risk of a repeat of the suicidal episode.

Distraction

Distraction can be a legitimate, conscious, intentional, and healthy strategy when a person is struggling with suicidal thoughts. When I was first learning this tool in the dialectical behavioral therapy (DBT) parent classes I had to take for my niece, it seemed ridiculous that in a suicidal crisis, the best move and the right thing to do might be watching a funny movie, or having a coloring session, or playing with the family pet. But in reality, getting through a bout of suicidal ideation (much like getting through many hard things in life) is truly often a matter of getting through this moment, and then the next moment and the next moment until you are . . . through.

Sometimes, our kids need us to help them access their toolboxes of things to do when they are upset or feeling suicidal. Whenever in my life I've felt down or depressed, I had many different actions I would take to get through those moments, many tools I could use to distract myself until the moments passed. But my niece started with an empty toolbox, and she often went straight to feeling suicidal when I and others might detour first through yelling, crying, watching tv, reading, calling friends, rage-cleaning, and ice cream, long before we ever might get to feeling suicidal. *(Except I would never rage-clean. Ice cream, yes. Toilet scrubbing, no.)* Some kids, whether because of mental health issues like anxiety or depression, or from trauma, or simply the mysteries of how we develop, just aren't equipped with these tools. Part of their recovery will be helping our kids discover for themselves what works for them, and then helping them practice using those tools in the moments when they need them.

Sometimes, our kids may be so dysregulated, so out of sorts, depressed or anxious, that before they can even watch a movie, or try anything else, they first need to just breathe, just literally breathe. Learn four to five breathing exercises and be ready to do them with your child. Teach them that breathing exercises can literally change the chemicals being secreted in their brain that are causing escalated anxiety or fearful feelings.

Other things to try when distraction is called for:

- Paint your nails
- Bake
- Journal
- Go for a walk, get out in nature
- Engage one or all of the five senses: smell something good; touch a fuzzy blanket; look at pictures that make you happy or memes that make you laugh; listen to a playlist of favorite music; taste your favorite cookie.
- Put together (if they haven't already either in the hospital or in therapy) a literal box of items that will help them be present to themselves, with many of the items above. They can use this toolbox when they need it.

- Sit under a weighted blanket

- Listen to poetry or scripture or music

- Call a friend

- Pet your cat or your dog

- Watch a movie

- Watch stand-up comedy, or whatever show or YouTube video is guaranteed to make them laugh

- Dance—crank up the playlist and dance like nobody's watching!

"Normal" household expectations

When your child is or recently has been in crisis, by necessity, family life begins to revolve around the child and the child's problems. This is natural and necessary, FOR A SHORT PERIOD OF TIME. It is not sustainable or healthy long-term, not for you, your child, or other family members.

Whenever you are not in urgent crisis, work hard to return your family to a state of functioning that accounts for everyone's needs. You will find a new household rhythm, and you will need to make it as normal as possible, for you, your child and any other kids at home.

I'm not saying this is easy. When you have one teenager who is dealing with active suicidal thoughts, and one who is largely doing fine, it can be tempting to treat chores, expectations, and behaviors differently. To be sure, there have been times when household expectations and fairness were temporarily suspended, and I'm sure there have been times when I let that go on too long.

Sometimes that makes sense, and certainly it's important for us to recognize legitimate limitations that our child or teen is experiencing because of their mental illness. But at the same time, it's important that your teen also learn that fair or not, they need to function around other people in spite of their illness, that they still need to be a team player, they still need to be kind, and whenever possible, they still need to empty the dishwasher and vacuum the stairs when it's their turn.

Just because your child is suicidal, doesn't mean that you must do everything they want the way they want. It does no one any good if they become the de facto ruler of the household because you are afraid that continuing to parent them reasonably and appropriately will result in a suicide.

But parenting gets real scary when the perceived *(or real? what if they're real?)* consequences of being too harsh/strict/demanding are not a normal surly teenager, but death.

Yep, that's the crux of it for some of us, isn't it? We're afraid that any wrong move and our kids will die. But we also worry about not asking enough of them, of enabling them to be entitled, of actually feeding their depression and hopelessness by not requiring them to get out and do their homework/go to school/get a job/put their freaking dishes in the dishwasher!

Normal expectations and responsibilities can help a child feel a sense of purpose within the family and remind them they are capable. Those are good things. Remember, your child is still the same person, and your family still has the same rules, values, and expectations.

At the same time, it's important for the rest of the family to accept that some limitations are legitimate, and being a compassionate family member means recognizing that and being okay with it.

It can be difficult for those of us who don't struggle with mental illness to realize just how variable a person's capacity can be, and how real that is. One day might be a good day, and they can do their chores, participate in family dinner, and do their homework. The next day might be a bad day, and all they can do is curl up in bed and watch videos. That's real, it stinks, it's not fair to them or anyone else, and that is the nature of mental illness.

Accepting and then accommodating that can be hard, but it's easier when you are talking to your child openly about how they are feeling and holding reasonable expectations for them while also being open to hard days.

What's the balance when it comes to household expectations? How do we live in that tension? Step by step, day by day, figuring it out as we go. Is that last sentence a cop-out because there is no easy answer? Yes, it is, AND you can trust yourself as a parent to do your best.

Next steps: being sure to get the right diagnosis, the right plan and the right treatment

Your child needs a complete and robust diagnosis as early as possible in their mental health journey, whether your child has been hospitalized for their suicidal ideation or not. Then, their treatment team should reevaluate the diagnosis as they age, and with any major changes in behavior or symptoms. A child who struggles with ADHD in elementary school, for instance, may develop severe depression as they enter puberty, or serious anxiety, and that will require a different treatment plan. Different therapeutic and medical treatments work differently, or more effectively, for kids as they age and go through new seasons in their life.

Treatment for various mental health conditions varies widely, but the proper treatment given improperly for the wrong issues can not only be ineffective, but can make things significantly worse.

Not only that, but not all therapists, pediatricians, or even psychiatrists are comfortable managing suicidality. It is critically important to keep looking until you find a team that is. This is not the time for an inexperienced or generalist provider. You need someone with a high comfort level, extensive education, and specific experience with kids who are suicidal.

It is important to factor in other conditions your child may live with, including types of neurodivergence such as ADHD or autism spectrum disorder. These can affect both the course of your child's mental health struggles, their ability to learn new skills and coping mechanisms, and the best approach to help them. Experiencing serious trauma will also affect their mental health journey and treatment, and it can also cause its own mental health problems, such as post-traumatic stress disorder.

If your child is suicidal for longer than just a brief, passing time, it is more likely that they are experiencing a serious mental illness. *(Am I saying they DO have a serious mental illness? No. That's why a thorough evaluation is so important. And let's be real. ANY mental illness that's happening to your child is serious.)*

If your child has an SMI, you are on a different level, a different battlefield. Therapy may be a part of the appropriate treatment regimen for your child, but it won't be everything.

Serious mental illnesses (SMI) such as major depressive disorder, bipolar disorder, schizophrenia and schizoaffective disorder, obsessive compulsive disorder (OCD), complex post-traumatic stress disorder (C-PTSD), and eating disorders such as anorexia require complex, brain-based medical care. It is generally not appropriate for these particular disorders to be treated solely with talk therapy.

Psychosis

If psychosis (delusions, hallucinations, disorganized thinking or movement) is present, these symptoms should be addressed early and aggressively, because early intervention for psychosis can make a HUGE difference in the course of your child's mental health. Early intervention works. (For more information, see resource section.)

I know that words like psychosis are scary. It is terrifying when your child is experiencing a break from reality. It's also terrifying to think about whether psychosis might mark the onset of a complicated condition such as schizophrenia. Getting a diagnosis is critical for determining whether the psychosis indicates the start of a chronic condition or is related to an acute illness or substance use. Some psychosis resolves with early identification and intervention.

I promise that ***the consequences of denial***—hoping the psychosis is just a phase or hoping you aren't seeing what you are seeing—***are scarier***. Knowledge is power, and taking well-informed action is the best way to get your child the help that they need. Remember, though, that even if your child has serious mental illness, there is hope, and recovery is possible! Even the most serious mental illness can respond to treatment, and people can better manage their disorder with the right help and support.

Parenting a suicidal child = making decisions you never thought you'd have to make

You ~~may~~ will find yourself having to make decisions you never thought you would make. One recent summer I was preparing to go to the National Speakers Association annual conference, the premier learning event for my field, when one night my daughter had a major suicidal episode that landed us back in the emergency room. We spent, as you do, a few hours there, talking with the doctor on call as well as the social worker. Hearing her cry hopelessly and tell the social worker that she just did not want to keep trying, she did not want to be alive anymore, was heartbreaking and scary.

Scary enough that I had the social worker nearly convinced that admission was necessary, even though we'd gotten a particularly grumpy, brusque gal who was much more inclined along the lines of "suck it up, hospitalization isn't treatment and it won't help."

But when she went out to see if beds were available, I checked back in with my daughter and we talked. I asked her what she thought she truly needed in that moment, and told her that I would support her no matter what.

By that point it was about 11:30 pm, and A said, "I just want to go home and go to bed." Then (because that's what you do as a mom/ parent/caregiver) I immediately second-guessed a bit, quizzed her hard about safety and got a pinkie promise that she would commit to a safety plan, take suicide off the table, and tell me if that changed.

So, we went home. (After talking again to the doctor and the social worker, of course, and waiting and waiting and waiting for the discharge paperwork, because that's an emergency room visit.)

And just a couple of days later, I got on a plane to go to my conference, leaving her with her fully capable, caring, and loving dad. Did I second-guess THAT decision? You bet. Did I call more often than normal, check in a (probably) annoying amount? Yep, sure did.

I never imagined that I would fly across the country just a couple of days after my child had had such a serious suicidal episode. However, when a person lives with severe depression and suicidal ideation, healing will come with bumps in the road. You will think you are doing okay, until you aren't. Then when you know things aren't okay, you will realize that you can't stay home by their side, arms around them, staring deeply into their eyes, forever. You communicate openly, make support plans, take a deep breath, and hope you are trusting your child in the right moment; and then, you have to go to work, get gas in the car, buy avocados, and live your life.

You also have to take care of yourself. That night in the emergency room was traumatic for me, excruciatingly difficult to hear. I was tired, emotionally drained, and not necessarily in the best mood for a professional learning opportunity in Florida. However, I also recognized that I needed the physical distance and the mental break. In fact, I extended my stay by a day to go to Disney World.

That's right. I went to Disney World, by myself, for a day, leaving an actively suicidal-ish teen at home.

Like I said, you will find yourself making some unbelievably difficult and/or strange decisions that you would never have anticipated making.

My choice to go ahead and take my trip was an intentional signal to my daughter: a signal that I trusted her; I believed in her ability to keep herself safe; and that a pinkie promise made, was a pinkie promise that must be kept.

Could it have all gone horribly wrong? Yes, of course. But the worst can happen if we're at home, too.

I was faced with a similar situation just about six months later. I had to fly to Alaska to be with a friend whose husband was having a serious medical crisis. We thought my daughter was doing well, and she'd had a decent spell of stability. But I got a call from my husband several days into my trip, letting me know that our daughter had walked into his office and given him all of her meds to hold because she was having a hard time and didn't think she should have them for a few days.

What!? We thought she was doing okay!? Nothing particular had happened, just the ~~natural normal~~ awful course of severe depression. But when you think everything is okay, and you find out that everything is most definitely NOT OKAY, it can be incredibly disconcerting. It's normal to question yourself and your parenting all over again, as I did, and wonder if you will ever believe that your child will ever REALLY be okay. *(BTW, I have no answer for that yet. I'll keep you posted.)*

In addition to questioning my parenting decisions, I questioned, and despaired for, my own future. I struggled with feeling like: "I'll never get a break, it will always be hard, I'm being punished for taking care of myself, what if the worst happens while I'm here? Will it be my fault? Will I be able to live with myself?" Then, of course, I struggled with guilt for even thinking about myself, and worrying about my own feelings.

I called my daughter and talked with her. She again assured me that although she wasn't good, she was safe, that she had checked in with her therapist, and she would be okay. My husband and I talked, and we decided that it wasn't necessary for me to come home. I worried, I prayed, I checked in too much, and I had to trust that they had it handled. Which they did.

None of that mattered that night when I still couldn't sleep, and when I did finally sleep, I woke up from a sound sleep to find myself in the midst of a full-blown panic attack. Have I mentioned how grateful I am for my therapist? No? Well, I am. This is HARD, y'all.

Hard Things to Remember When Unexpected Bumps Happen

- This downswing, this moment, is a bump. It isn't a new forever reality. It is part of the healing process, it's normal, and it's not permanent. *(Maybe I should have that set to music so we can sing it to ourselves.) (It is shocking how quickly our minds can spiral on this.)*

- If you **know** your child is having a bad time, that's a GOOD thing. It means they are talking to you, and open with you. Again, that's a GOOD thing.

- Remember, the things your child says in a downswing are also not reality, and they are not permanent. Those statements— like the difficult things my daughter shared in the emergency room—are mental illness talking, and the mental illness lies. Try and think of them like things a toddler says during a tantrum. Not to minimize your child's pain, or their feelings, but they are temporary. *(Let's keep that analogy to ourselves, shall we? I think it makes a good point, but I also think it would be ILL-ADVISED to compare your teen's suicidal statements to a temper tantrum. ILL-ADVISED. Not helpful.)*

- Short of actual physical threat or injury, don't panic. *(At least not on the outside.)* Use these bumps to practice your new skills and your child's new skills. Calmly act in the same way you would if your child commonly has asthma attacks, or diabetes, or flares of any other serious or chronic illness.

- Take care of yourself. Their bumps are your bumps too, so you will BOTH need extra rest, grace and love.

A story, and a caution about parental denial

Remember how in the beginning of the book I talked about how there were no chapters about this in the baby books? You do not know how to parent a suicidal child because really, no one has that all worked out. It's hard, it's nebulous, it's scary, and there are no perfect answers or approaches.

You will make mistakes. You might make colossal mistakes, **because you are human and this is hard** and no one knows exactly how to do it right and you are doing the best you can. I know we were, when we made what was almost the worst mistake of our parenting lives.

To be honest, I didn't want to write this story; I don't want you or anyone else to know how dumb we were. But I'm sharing it to say that we all can screw up, and so you don't make the same mistakes we did, mistakes that could easily have cost us our child. Approximately eight months after her hospital stay, our daughter A was in her first semester of college. We knew she was struggling with classes and academics, and that was worrisome, but we thought everything was generally ok. But it wasn't. Her depression wasn't well controlled, and she called us one night and asked us to come get her because she didn't feel safe to herself. As it turns out, she had very nearly made a suicide attempt, had nearly chosen to overdose on the medications she had in her dorm room.

Of course we brought her home. We discussed whether she felt like she needed to go to the ER again (she didn't feel like that was necessary), and we stayed close. We watched movies, we hung out, we talked a little bit but not too much. She had a call the next day with her psychiatrist, who was shocked because he'd thought things were better too. The doctor recommended either withdrawing from school—at least for the semester—or continuing to go to school while living at home, which would have been inconvenient though theoretically doable. She refused. Flat refused. She declared that she was sure that if she didn't go back, she'd feel like even more of a failure. And she would definitely kill herself.

Was that true? Was it 18-year-old melodrama? How could we tell? Did it matter?

We went along with it. We talked about a safety plan, we met with the on-campus disabilities coordinator *(as mental health issues fit under the disabilities umbrella, and the coordinator was SO helpful and kind)*, and we made agreements to check in with each other twice a day at least. We thought—in our worry and confusion and, at the same time, our attempts to honor our child's autonomy and her ability to self-manage her mental health *(after all, she had reached out to us and was open when she was in crisis)*—we thought we'd checked all of the boxes.

Those weren't bad impulses or intentions, they weren't. After all, for many of our kids, these mental health struggles may last for a long time and may even be something they struggle with their whole lives. They **do** need to learn to be in charge of their mental health and what they can and cannot handle. *(This is obviously different when talking about someone who has psychosis or other breaks with reality and the ability to reason, in which case they may truly not know what they can and cannot handle.)*

So where did we screw up? When we drove her back to college, we drove her back and left her with all of her medications—the same medications she had nearly overdosed on just days earlier. We dropped her off at her dorm, the dorm room she didn't even share with a roommate, with all of those medications.

Why did we do that? I don't know. I know that when I relayed to a friend the next day, who was also a mental health expert and author, what we had done, my friend was so upset with me and scared for my kid that she was actually angry. Her helpless anger helped me get clear real quick. Needless to say, I immediately drove the hour back to campus and retrieved all but a week's worth of medication, and for the rest of the semester drove out each week to deliver the next week's worth. *(Note: you should know how much of your child's medication is fatal, and during times such as this, make sure they have access to less than that. I'm sorry, that's dark, but also important.)*

Would she have been okay if we didn't? Maybe. But that's the worst decision we've knowingly made in this season, and we could have lost her because of it.

Except that we wouldn't have truly lost her because of that choice. We would have lost her because of major depression. We would have lost her because of an impulsive choice she would have made in a hopeless moment of pain. Remember, no matter what happens with your child, you can't be with them every minute, and you can't prevent someone who is truly intent on taking their own life from doing it. All you can do is the best you can do in that moment.

Is that how I would truly feel if the worst had happened? I hope so, but maybe not. I'm human too.

· · · · · · · ·

Why did we make that initial, clearly terrible choice? I really, truly don't know, not entirely. But if forced to explain, I think that the closest I can come is to reference the deep, deep tendency of a parent to be in denial, to act as if this isn't a life-threatening medical emergency, and to minimize the situation because it is so damn terrifying. *(Even if you are an expert on mental health, a speaker and author on the subject! Denial is real, and powerful!)*

We act as if things aren't that bad, because we deeply don't want them to be that bad, when they ARE CLEARLY THAT BAD.

Recognizing our extraordinary capacity for denial as parents is difficult, but necessary. It's a first step to guarding against that denial, and making better, more informed decisions for our kids.

Stay present

What are you feeling?

Fear
Anxiety
Isolated
Panicked
Guilty
Sad
Lonely
Ashamed
Frustrated
Angry
Hopeless
Grieving
Questioning
Inadequate
Helpless
Exhausted

I'm going to ask you to take just a minute right now, or a couple of minutes, to do a self-assessment. Get present to this moment. Take note of yourself, how you are feeling, what you are feeling.

You may not be a person who takes much stock in or spends much time paying attention to your own feelings. If so, right now you are probably impatiently rolling your eyes at me and wishing I'd get on with it. I get it, because I'm married to someone like that *(and I love him)*.

But here's the deal—if you aren't self-aware, you aren't going to be as effective as you can be for your child. Your "stuff" is going to get in the way more than necessary, and that's not optimal. So, humor me.

If, on the other hand, you are a person *(such as myself)* for whom **Feelings Are Life,** if you are all about your feelings and sometimes overwhelmed by your feelings, then you need to take a moment as well. Again, your "stuff" is going to get in the way more than necessary, and that's not optimal.

When you are caring for a person with suicidal thoughts, you need to be as calm, clear-headed, reassuring, and confident as possible. *(There is a chance that the impossible nature of that statement might trigger hysterical laughter. I would tell you to stop laughing, but honestly, laughter is super healthy and a decent strategy for helping you to achieve a physical state of calm and clear-headed, so go ahead and laugh.)*

Just for a moment, take note of yourself.

· · · · · · ·

Start with breathing. If you are reading this book, it stands to reason that it may have been a while since you've done any truly healthy breathing. When we are stressed, or scared, or anxious, we tend to breath shallowly.

Shallow breaths actually tell our bodies and our nervous system that we should continue to feel stressed, scared and anxious, which then makes us breathe more shallowly, which causes our nervous systems . . . you get it. Again, that's not optimal.

Stopping to take even two or three slow, calm breaths will literally change your brain's chemical signaling, and positively affect your nervous system. Do that, now: take three slow, deep breaths.

Now, what are you feeling?

Fear
Anxiety
Isolated
Panicked
Guilty
Sad
Lonely
Ashamed
Frustrated
Angry
Hopeless
Grieving
Questioning
Inadequate
Helpless
Exhausted

Normal. All of those things are normal, rational responses to what you are going through, whether you are feeling them one at a time, or all at once, or some combination of them in dizzying rotating fashion. Those are completely normal ways to feel about an impossibly difficult situation.

So if you have wasted *even three seconds* feeling bad about feeling bad, **STOP IT**. You don't have time for that, and you don't have the emotional bandwidth for that.

Just accept that, for now, you are feeling what you are feeling. Call it out for what it is. Once you recognize how you are feeling, you are at least more capable of taking proactive steps to deal with it in a way that doesn't negatively impact your child, or your relationship with your child.

In a later section I'll share my philosophy of self-care for the caregiver, and some ideas that you can and should try, but in the meantime, acknowledge how you're feeling, and tell yourself that it's okay. It really is.

By the way, I think pretty much *every* entry on that list, every type of feeling you might be feeling, all boils down to fear. Fear. You are afraid of losing your child. Of course you are. That's okay.

I believe that managing our fear is both the biggest obstacle for parents of suicidal kids, and also the biggest opportunity we have to become the best parents we can be. The key to managing that fear?

Practicing staying in the present moment, with your child and for your child. A parent who can stay present can think more clearly and make better decisions, they can be more emotionally available and effective for their child, and they can best manage the natural, normal fear they have about possibly losing their child.

Allowing that fear to run amok means you lose your ability to stay in the present moment. Managing that fear, no matter how difficult it is, prevents you from panicking, from overreacting, and from overwhelming your child. Because you don't have time for any of that.

Oh, and you know what else you don't have time for? You don't have time for wondering if this is your fault because you let them watch too much TV when they were little, or you had that one piece of soft brie when you were pregnant, or because depression or some other mental illness runs in your family.

It. Doesn't. Matter. So, STOP IT.

What matters is that you are reading this book now, you care about your child, you love them, and want them to be well and you are doing the best you can.

Just keep doing the best you can. That's okay, too.

Mindfulness isn't just woo woo

How do you learn to manage your fear and stay in the present moment? One of the most effective ways you can learn to stay present is to learn and practice mindfulness.

I don't know what your reaction is when someone talks about mindfulness. If you are one of those people who immediately pictures a hippie yoga instructor hypnotically suggesting that you become one with the ants and the grass and the Earth Spirit while she plays a harp with her toes, I get it.

Mindfulness gets lumped in with many New Age approaches to life, such as crystals, shamanic journeys, and astrology, and, in fact, each of those may have their uses. *(OK, honestly, I don't see it cause it's not my thing, but if that's your thing, you do you. Go with your bad self.)*

But in all seriousness, there is nothing woo woo about the discipline of mindfulness. Mindfulness is a choice, a trainable practice, and evidence-based science. Cultivating mindfulness will not only help you and your child better manage difficult situations physically and mentally, but it will also GUARANTEE you more time with those you love.

That may sound like a particularly bold claim, but it's simple math. We spend an inordinate amount of time each day fretting and thinking about the past, and scheming and worrying about the future. Think about how many times a day your mind drifts back to a difficult moment with your child or contentious conversation that happened at work; and how many times you find yourself imagining the worst possibilities for the future. Take every single one of those moments, and ask the following two questions:

- Did your time and your thoughts alter the past or change the future? *(I'm going to guess no, unless the future you were worrying about was a runaway bus imminently hurtling toward you and you were planning to jump aside. In which case, well done.)*

- During the moment in which you were thinking about the past or the future, were you completely focused on who or what was directly in front of you?

(Again, no. It's simply not possible for your brain to fully BE in more than one place/topic/moment at a time. It's not possible. Humans cannot do it.)

Every moment of the day that you spend thinking about the past or worrying about the future is a minute in which you do not bring your best self to the people around you, and in fact in many of those moments you are so disconnected from the people and events around you that you are merely functioning on autopilot.

Do these scenarios sound familiar?

"How in the world did I get home? I drove but I don't remember one thing about the drive."

"Mom, Mom? Mom! You aren't listening to me!"

You weren't present to those moments. You were mentally elsewhere.

· · · · · · ·

I'm not trying to make you feel guilty. I'm trying to help you see how critical this is because it's so easy to ignore. Nor am I claiming it's easy, and let's face it, sometimes it's convenient. *(Hellooooo, weekly staff meeting. Also, hellooooo, your child's 14th update today on* Fortnite *or* Pokémon. *Strategic zoning out can be helpful.)*

Mindfulness is simply the practice of keeping yourself aware and present to the only moment you are **guaranteed** to live, the one you are in right now.

Why do you need to constantly nurture mindfulness? Because it can be tempting to be anywhere in our minds but here, especially when here is difficult. When you have a suicidal child, there is a LOT to worry about, and probably many past moments you will be tempted to relive out of regret, frustration or trauma. Human brains are distractible, skittish, avoidant of difficulty, and prone to wasting time and energy worrying about the future or agonizing and perseverating over the past.

Being mindful is a courageous choice.

· · · · · · ·

I came to realize that I needed to stay present to and embrace the silly version of my niece, K, who showed up in the evenings, chatty and funny, or obsessed with crime shows. I needed to stay present to the moments when she played with my little ones, and when she helped clean the kitchen.

Honestly, there were many periods of time when I wasn't sure K was going to survive long enough to heal. There were years in which it was entirely possible that K's suicidal ideation, her PTSD, and depression might prove to be fatal.

I realized that I wanted her to know she was deeply loved even if the worst happened, and she did not survive. I further realized that the only way I could be sure she knew she was loved was if I could stay present with her, in the right-now, the only moments I was guaranteed. If I could do that, then she would know she was loved.

She would know she was loved.

Her mental illness, her childhood trauma, her deep depression and horrible PTSD? I couldn't control any of that.

But staying present to my moments with her, and making sure she knew she was loved? THAT was in my control.

That reasoning alone—melodramatic though it is—makes staying mindful important. There are also other significant benefits to practicing mindfulness. Whether you think of what you are doing as prayer, meditation, or simply cultivating stillness and awareness, regular focus on mindfulness powerfully benefits our physical health, lowering blood pressure, decreasing depression and anxiety, and bringing necessary rest to your sympathetic nervous system. This is the part of the nervous system that is activated during danger or crisis, fight or flight.

Living with a suicidal teenager, and in fact BEING a suicidal teenager, is a traumatic experience, and trauma will mess with your sympathetic nervous system. After days, weeks or months of being hypervigilant, anxious, and exhausted, you or your child will likely become overly activated, and you may need to employ tools and techniques to help yourself settle, allow yourself to relax.

· · · · · · ·

There are many resources for learning and practicing mindfulness, and aside from a few basic suggestions, I will leave you to research more. I would highly recommend classes or videos on breathing techniques; yoga classes; any faith practices that resonate with you, such as prayer or meditation; and meditative physical activity such as walking. *(Or, if you're into that sort of thing, running. I most definitely am not, unless angry bears are involved, but people who run tell me it's helpful for mindfulness.)*

But wait, WHY, why did this happen?

Still stuck on the why?

Two things:

1. Understand that **right now, it doesn't matter why they feel suicidal.** It **is** how they feel, it is what they are experiencing right now, and the why of it can be *(and don't get me wrong, it should be)* dealt with later.

2. **It's not your fault.** I know I've already said this, but there is zero positive benefit to worrying about whether your child's suicidal ideation is your fault. I believe that the very fact that you are reading this book right now means you want the best for your child, you care about them, and you are willing to learn and implement new approaches to help them heal.

If you are in a situation in which you or your child are being abused, then get help immediately.

If that does not describe you, then right now you need to focus on helping your child heal. If there are factors in your family or your parenting that have contributed to your child's mental health struggles, you can address those moving forward, but really, none of us are perfect. We come into parenting with our own experience of how we were parented, our own resources or lack thereof, and our own immediate circumstances.

Let's be honest, there is a truth to the common joke among parents that we should all be saving for our children's future therapy fund, but we are all doing the best we can. You are doing the best you can.

Mental health struggles happen to everyone, at all stages of life, from all walks of life, all socioeconomic levels. It doesn't matter if you are rich, if you're struggling to pay the bills, if this has never happened to anyone in your family before *(unlikely, by the way. It did, they just didn't used to talk about this stuff)*, or if you took all of the parenting classes and did all of the things. Mental illness, including depression, anxiety, bipolar disorder, schizophrenia, etc., can and does happen in all families. No one is immune. It's part of the human experience.

Stop wasting your very limited energy on the "why." For right now, stay present, love your kid, and get them the help they need.

Communicate Openly

Start by asking your child

Getting through this season with your child will require open communication from everyone involved. Between you and your child, between your child and their mental health providers, and between you and your spouse or partner if you have one.

But effective, open communication is a skill, and may not be one that you and your child have practiced. How do you start?

> ASK YOUR CHILD HOW THEY ARE FEELING
> AND WHAT THEY NEED. THEN LISTEN.

You're more likely to get it right, it's respectful and caring, you give them some autonomy, and you let them know you trust and expect them to take an active, responsible role in their recovery.

And—I remember how incredulous and mad I was, when I realized how much of the tactical approach to my niece's recovery would be based on her own self reporting.

It seemed like a terrible system! It made no sense. Why are we depending on children who are suicidal to tell us whether they are really suicidal, just a little suicidal, or a mere modicum of suicidal? For crying out loud, they're children! They're suicidal children!

Sometimes, suicidal people LIE about their feelings so they can be freer to make an attempt, or prepare for one *(K did)*, or just to get their parents off their back so they can keep playing *Minecraft*. This can't possibly be the approach, the best way to assess their risk day to day. Just *ask* them? Really?

But it's true, which I've rediscovered as we walk this road with A. When A came home from the hospital, the doctor recommended that we continue to check in each day, and come up with and agree to a way to get a daily assessment of where A was in terms of depression, anxiety, and suicidal thoughts.

Parents need to practice and get comfortable asking about the intensity of how their kid is feeling, saying it. One way to do that is to have your child name the intensity on a scale of 1-10, after defining the scale themselves.

We settled with A on a scale of 1-10, so at a minimum, and hopefully without being too annoying, I can just ask "how are your numbers today?" A may say, 5, 4 and 2, or 4, 7 and 7, for instance, and if none of the numbers are too high, we don't have to have any other long discussions.

How do we know if the numbers are too high? Which numbers, specifically, are too high? What do we do if the numbers **are** too high? There are no magic numbers and no magic answers. Remember how we've talked about using your best judgment, listening to your gut, looking them in eye and doing the best you can with the info you have? Yeah, that. Sorry.

However, in a situation in which you are using a scale like this, 1-10, ask your child in a good moment to tell you a little bit more about what different numbers mean to them, and when they think you should be concerned. Let them know you trust them to tell you what they need, and when they need more help.

We all tend to operate on self-report. How do I feel? How should that affect my actions? What do I do with how I feel?

Best case scenario, isn't that what their whole life will be? In fact, if your child learns now how to track and respond to their own internal emotional state, and to regulate even under difficult circumstances, in the future they will be that much stronger for themselves and everyone around them.

We have to trust them first

The hard truth is we have to begin to trust them before they can learn to trust themselves. Ouch. Agonizingly difficult, I know, but it's true. To trust them, we need to communicate, and by communicate, I mean listen.

This is a skill we can help our kids learn, and it may also be a skill that we need to grow within ourselves, too. Because many of us were raised with parents who were much more about telling and much less about listening, even if they were amazing, loving parents. That certainly described my parents' approach, and described the way I initially parented my own kids. You do what you know, right? *(This is an important point to remind yourself about, to give yourself grace about, and even to forgive yourself for on the regular.)*

You can begin by practicing this even with smaller issues, to help both you and your kid learn to communicate openly and learn to trust each other.

For instance, after a rough day at school, or when something is obviously wrong, my friend Leanne will ask her kids, who both have significant mental health struggles: do you need a snack, do you need to talk about it, or do you need a nap? I mean honestly, none of us stray too far from those basic preschool age needs, do we?

This approach is brilliant for a few reasons. It tells your child that you respect their autonomy. It gives them the message that you believe that they know what they need and you are there to help them get what they need. Finally, it places mental health days squarely in the same bucket as bad physical health days, which is exactly where they should be.

(Note: If your child has lack of insight because they are experiencing serious mental illness like bipolar or psychosis, that will definitely complicate

your communication. But being non-threatening, comforting and compassionate is still going to be your best approach.)

It's OK to ask them

Asking your child, or anyone, if they are having suicidal thoughts, is NOT going to make them more likely to be suicidal or to act on those thoughts. Asking will make it more likely they will feel supported, loved, and seen. It can help them feel supported and strong enough to ask for help, and to follow through with getting help if they need it. In fact, asking your child directly if they are planning to kill themselves can be the best way to prevent them from killing themselves!

If you're reading this book, you've probably already had some sort of conversation about suicide with your child, but if you haven't or if it still makes you nervous, I just want to reassure you that you will not make it worse by asking directly or speaking openly about their suicidal thoughts.

As one expert shared with me, "In the end, we don't and can't control someone else's behavior. All we can do is create a relationship and an environment in which we can be honest and direct—I need to hear what you are thinking; are you thinking about suicide?"

In fact, by asking directly, you let your child know that you are a safe person they can talk to about these very scary thoughts, that you don't need them to protect you from their scary thoughts, and that you aren't going to panic. Rather than freaking out when your child shares their thoughts about suicide, do everything in your power to remain curious. Your child has been brave and real with you. If you freak out, they will shut down, and there will be a higher chance in the future that you WILL NOT KNOW WHAT IS REALLY GOING ON.

("Let's be real" addendum—You probably will freak out, at least once, and while it may not be helpful, it is pretty normal. Just apologize, tell them you're working on it, and you'll do better. Then try and do better.)

Suicidal thoughts can not only be scary to the person having them, but they can even begin to feel like they have their own powers. Seeing your calm response to their scary thoughts can help take the magical power away from those thoughts.

It's also okay, and recommended, that you ask them if they have a specific plan for ending their life, and if they have access to ways to actually carry it out. Have they thought about exactly how they would kill themself? Do they have a plan? Do they have access to the means to carry that plan out? All of this is important information to help you and medical providers monitor your child's level of risk.

(Also, if they say yes, then you need to remove all items that might be a risk—all pills, including OTC, knives, razors, guns, ropes, belts, poisons, etc.—from their environment. Remember, teens are impulsive at best, and it's our job to make sure they don't have easy access to ways to hurt themselves.)

Be detectives together

One of your most important jobs in your child's learning journey will be helping them learn to be their own best advocate. To do that, you both need to become detectives. You need to be a detective of your child, and you need to teach them to be their own detective for their own mental health. This is a concept I learned from my author friend Julie Fast, and I think it is super helpful.

What does it mean to be a detective of your mental health? It means paying attention, making observations, drawing conclusions and testing those conclusions, and then making more observations. A good mental health detective (of their own mental health or on behalf of a child or loved one) will take note of:

- History—what is their history of mental health behaviors and symptoms?

- Triggers—what makes them feel worse?

- Look back and take note of what things have worked to keep them safe in the past—what makes them feel better?

- What can they do to distract themselves during hard moments?

- If distraction doesn't work, what other activities help them self-regulate (example: take a shower)?
- If those things don't work, who are the people and what are the spaces they need to be safe?

Once these observations are tracked and noted, the next step is to practice and test what you've learned, continue to make observations, and tweak and adjust as necessary. It is also important for your child to learn and practice effectively communicating these observations to a doctor or other provider.

· · · · · · ·

When our kids are little, we can tell them when to go to bed, what shows to watch, and what medicine to take and when. But as kids get older, we need to help them learn to trust themselves, and trust that they know what they need while as a parent we are still setting boundaries. *(Because no one NEEDS to play* Fortnite *all night every night.)*

Focus on and equip your child to decide for themselves what can create safety for them now and in the future. The goal is to get stronger in as many places as we can, because we don't control life. As parents we need to take a collaborative approach with our child, defining problems and finding help that will work for them.

The Big Goal

The overall goal of helping someone manage suicidal thoughts is to directly affect and expand the space between the suicidal thought and the ability to actually make an attempt. This can mean physical barriers, barriers of time and space, or barriers of emotional anchors that prevent your child from acting on a suicidal plan. Be a detective with your child, and decide what suicidal thoughts mean for THEM, and what an appropriate response to those thoughts might be.

As you and your child move forward in their healing journey, you may well need to come to a place where you calmly accept expressions of suicidal thoughts, especially if they are an ongoing or longstanding issue with your child. Your child and their team may decide that suicidal thoughts do not automatically qualify as a crisis that results in you throwing your child in the car and driving to the closest ER. Instead, you will learn that the response to those thoughts needs to be specific to your child, and one that you and their team help them develop for themselves.

Help your child observe, catalog, and categorize:

- What does your brain say in those moments?

- What thoughts start to pop up more frequently?

- What behaviors start happening for you that are red flags?

Together, you, your child, and their team will all decide when it IS time for the emergency room, and when the appropriate steps are instead distraction, or close monitoring, or a walk in the park, or practicing some other coping skill that gets them through to the next moment. In calm moments, you can ask, "If I see X behavior, what can I do that is most helpful?" or "If I hear you say Y, what do you need that would be most helpful?" Then the ideas you come up with together can be added to the safety plan.

NOTE: if you have gotten to this point in the book but the very idea of not treating suicidal thoughts as an emergency is horrifying to you, I get it. I really do. Early on I assumed that those thoughts would ALL have to be an emergency by their inherent nature. In reality, many people struggle with those thoughts on an ongoing basis, and healing means learning to cope with those thoughts without acting on them. HOWEVER, this is obviously a tricky area that you will ONLY act on in concert with your child's team. Every person and every child is so different, and you'll need to follow the entire team's direction for your child.

When you and your child can openly communicate, and you are both working to be good detectives of their mental health, you will both begin to understand your child's "normal" baseline. If in fact suicidal thoughts are a near daily occurrence, then that is their baseline, and maybe the danger point is only when they begin to make a plan and scheme how to carry out that plan.

But if your child has never before had a suicidal thought, the sudden appearance of mere suicidal thoughts may be a significant enough departure from their baseline to warrant emergency intervention.

When you've established a solid partnership with your child, both of you working as detectives of their mental health, then you will begin to have a more complete picture of what they need, the strength of their executive functioning skills, and their level of maturity and problem-solving. This knowledge will help you make good, nonjudgmental decisions for their safety.

For instance, knowing exactly when it is safe to unlock medications or return them to an older teen isn't easy. Same thing when it comes to knowing when it is okay to give them back their razors. These are tricky moments that will become easier as you, your child, and their treatment team practice open communication, and as they develop trust in themselves and in you.

So, now what? What do you do? What do they do? How do you know what is OK?

Short, unhelpful answer: there are no right answers to those questions.

AND it was exactly these types of questions that inspired me to write this book for you, and for all families whose loved one's struggle with suicidal thoughts.

"Mom, can I go hang out with my friends this afternoon?" My middle child was two days out from a particularly scary bout of suicidal ideation one week during her first semester of college. We'd brought her home, she'd gotten some sleep, we'd hung out in the living room and watched TV. She *seemed* better, she *said* she was better, and now she wanted some normalcy, and to hang out with some friends.

Was she really better? Was she being honest with me? Was this just a temporary upswing in her depression, relief that the scary moment had passed? Or *(whispered the scared mom voice in my head)* was she plotting to leave the house, and our supervision to more easily attempt suicide?

These are the types of day-to-day questions you may struggle to answer with your teen after every suicidal episode. How close do you keep them, for how long, and when do you know they are safe again?

Another short, unhelpful answer: remember in the very first chapter of this book, when I told you that you cannot save your child, and you cannot absolutely guarantee their safety even if you do all of the right things? Well, yeah, that.

There will always be uncertainty as you and your family make these decisions and live out these moments in your teen's journey. You will hold that uncertainty in one hand, while in the other hand you'll hold onto the best practices, advice and tips you can find.

It is not protective to prevent your child from being around their friends and instead keep them home with you. That is only an illusion of control. For adolescents, friends are sometimes more important to their emotional wellbeing than their parents, so we shouldn't deprive them of that health and safety factor. Friends can be as healing for a teen as their mental health providers as well. It's true for all of us, really, that our natural support networks are as/more important than professional therapeutic support, so as parents we shouldn't resist this. *(Obviously, if your child's friends are not safe, if there are concerns about substance use or other problematic behaviors, you will need to consider this more thoughtfully.)*

For my family, it often came down to safety plans, compromises, serious pinky swears, and direct conversation, building off of a history of direct conversations in which my child and my husband and I had previously built trust and understanding.

Be ready for when hard things happen

Talk openly about and be aware of triggers that might resurface your child's suicidal thoughts, things like major loss, including a breakup or a death; bullying or public humiliation; chronic or severe medical problems; and substance use or abuse.

Talk to your child when these events happen, help them anticipate potential difficulties, and plan how they would use their tools to protect themselves. Watch them extra closely, and check in more often,

Checking in: don't make it about you

Try to agree in advance on a way to check in with them that won't be too annoying. They may be teenagers, after all. "Are you doing okay?" is too open ended, and allows for the dreaded yes or no responses. Maybe "Mind if I check in right now about how you're doing? What's going well for you today? What isn't going well?"

Be careful of using language that tells your child **not** to be honest with you, or that encourages them to protect YOU. They can tell when you are asking a question for the purpose of seeking comfort and relief from your own anxiety. *(Sorry, but it's true.)* Watch out for and avoid questions like: "You're not feeling suicidal, are you?" or "You are feeling safe, right?" Questions like that immediately telegraph both your fear and your desired response, and your kid will immediately see your concern and your desire to be reassured. They may feel responsible for protecting your feelings, and then they will change their response to keep you from worrying or being scared. That's not good for you or for them.

As I've said before, we don't want our kids to feel like they need to hide how they feel in order to protect us, or make them responsible for reassuring us. We want to ask TRULY honest open-ended questions that give them full permission to be open with us, because we are the grownups, and we can handle their big and potentially scary feelings. If we're having a hard time with that *(and who wouldn't?!?)* we'll have to figure out how to take care of our emotional needs ourselves. (See Chapter: Take Care of Yourself.)

Remember, your job is to reassure them:

- it's okay to not be okay.

- nothing will shock you *(fake it with everything you've got if you have to)*.
- you can hear whatever it is they need to say.
- you can handle it, and you'll be okay.

If we allow our kids to feel responsible for our feelings, they will not be honest with us about their suicidal thoughts and plans. I know I'm repeating myself, but that's because this is incredibly hard for parents to do effectively.

I still caught myself, after years of practice with my nieces, asking my daughter if she was okay. When she said she was, I didn't fully believe her anyway, so why was I torturing us both? Sigh. I'm still working on it because it's that important.

Please hear me. Really check in with yourself. **It cannot be their job to make you feel better.**

Instead of:
"You're not feeling suicidal, are you?"

Try:
"Are you having active suicidal thoughts?"

Or

"How are the suicidal thoughts today, on a scale of 1-10?"

Or

"How are you doing, really?"

If it makes you feel any better, know that I STILL struggle with this. I am VERY good at asking questions that not-so-subtly point to the answer I'm hoping for. Real subtle ones, like "so, are you feeling good?" instead of just "how are you feeling, really?" We're a work in progress, just like our kids.

How do I know if they *really* mean it?

If you are still not sure if your suicidal child is serious, if you are not sure whether or not they are really in danger of taking their own life or if they are just "looking for attention," this section is for you, and I would encourage you to keep reading.

If you are quite sure your child is serious, and you already believe that the risk is real, you can totally skip this section. In fact, I would recommend it. The last thing you need right now is the amount of real that I am about to get up in here. In other words, I am about to get really real.

But if you are still reading because you are concerned that your child might be "just" seeking attention, or "just" trying to manipulate you, and you aren't sure how to respond, hear this. IT DOESN'T MATTER.

What if your child *isn't* actually serious about taking their life, but whatever things they've said, or told their therapist or their friend or a teacher, or the actions they've taken that have prompted you to read this book, really *are* "just" cries for help, or methods of seeking attention? *(This seems to be a frequent theme of unsolicited, outside input from family members and friends, and we can get really hung up here. See the next sentence.)*

IT DOESN'T MATTER.

If they've said things serious enough to make you or someone else wonder if they are in danger of hurting themselves, that's not okay. If you are wondering if your child is trying to manipulate you, think of it this way: If they are behaving in such a dangerous way just to manipulate you, that in and of itself is behavior in need of serious attention, so it doesn't matter. It's not healthy, and it means that your child is in need of serious intervention. Because a healthy, stable person who is not at risk wouldn't say or do things that would make other people think that they are.

The good news is that the appropriate thing to do in *either* case, whether they are in danger or trying to get attention, is to take it seriously and get them immediate psychiatric care. We as parents don't have to worry about perfectly parsing out how serious our kids might be in this situation, because the very act of talking about suicide means a child should be taken seriously, and taking them seriously will never be the wrong thing to do.

TAKING THEM SERIOUSLY WILL NEVER BE THE WRONG THING TO DO.

Your friends, your parents, the grandparents, someone at church might tell you that you need to just ignore your child, they are just trying to get attention and if you give it to them, it will only make things worse. These voices are messages from our recent cultural past, and the way we were often parented. If these are the messages that you hear in your head or from others, don't beat yourself up; it's natural that you might hear these old-school echoes. What's important is that you recognize that line of thinking will definitely not help, and it very well could make things worse.

Not only that, but teenagers are impetuous and impulsive. One moment they may just be intending to make a statement or trying to get your attention, and in the very next moment they might feel hopeless enough, or in enough pain, that they go ahead and attempt to hurt themselves.

Again, for the readers in the back . . . .

TAKING THEM SERIOUSLY WILL NEVER BE THE WRONG THING TO DO.

Every two hours in this country, a young person dies by suicide, according to the U.S. Centers for Disease Control (CDC). Every two hours. One in five teenagers will seriously consider suicide this year. Tragically, some of those young people had loved ones who did not believe they were serious, who did not want to "give in" to a kid who was seeking attention, and eighty percent of people who die by suicide gave verbal or nonverbal warning signs ahead of time.

For the love—and the life—of your child, give them the attention.

My niece made several overdose attempts over the years. The fact that the attempts were not fatal had nothing to do with how serious she felt, or whether this was just a cry for help or attention. The attempts were never fatal because of a mysterious combination of luck, her lack of knowledge about what might actually be fatal, and the hand of God. Sometimes she used ineffectual over-the-counter drugs, sometimes medications she'd been hoarding instead of swallowing, and once she used random pills given to her at a bus stop by a complete stranger. *(OK, and once she swallowed several of the tiny little bags of desiccant that you find in boxes of new shoes. It's OK to get a chuckle out of that. I did then and I do now. Sometimes a little dark humor is OK.)* Usually, either nothing happened or she felt gross, and/or she "just" had to have her stomach pumped.

Once, though, she had to have her stomach pumped and she still spent hours unresponsive, nearly in a coma, with kidney problems and heart irregularities. Yes, teenagers can be that dumb/risky/dangerous to themselves.

You have nothing to lose by taking them seriously, and frankly, possibly everything to lose by not taking them seriously.

Everything. To. Lose.

Real enough?

Feel free to share this chapter with Grandpa, or Aunt Judy, or whomever is getting into your head and making you question yourself. Because you ain't got time for that. So all together now:

TAKING THEM SERIOUSLY WILL NEVER BE THE WRONG THING TO DO.

TIPS FOR TALKING TO YOUR TEEN ABOUT MENTAL HEALTH

- Normalize mental illness by talking about it, because they already are! Mental health might be private, but it's not secret or shameful. Treat it like any other health issue, and discuss your family mental health history openly.

- Main lesson – by talk, I mostly mean LISTEN.

- Try to just be QUIET.

- Be curious, and don't assume you know what they are going through.

- Don't rush to reassure or tell them what they are feeling is silly or explain how they are wrong, EVEN if it's out of love and the need to make them (and you) feel better.

- Do your best not to overreact. If your teen feels they need to protect your feelings they will be less likely to share with you. Assure them that even thoughts about things like suicide, while scary, are normal, and you will work with them to get help.

When you DO talk – Helpful phrases to use:

- I wonder . . .

- Help me understand . . .

- That sounds hard/sad/difficult/scary. Tell me more . . .

- How would you like it to turn out?

- What can we do to get there?

- "How can I best support you right now?" instead of "Everything will be fine, you're okay, it's not as bad as you think"

- It's scary to hear you talk this way; I'm going to need more information.

Remember, you don't have to fix it—the suicidal thoughts, the overwhelming emotions, or the symptoms of mental illness. Sometimes being heard, loved, and understood really is enough, because you're validating how they feel right now. Validation means hearing, recognizing and acknowledging that your child's feelings are understandable, that you get where they are coming from, or how they might have come to feel the way they feel. It also means you are taking them seriously; you are understanding their behavior within the context of their life circumstances; you accept them; and that you have found the "kernel of truth" in their communication.

When you can find that kernel of truth in what they are saying or feeling, and let them know you hear them, it can take all of the air out of a tense or angry moment with your kid. Everyone wants to know they are heard and seen, and that the person they are with is trying to understand them.

When kids feel validated, they are better able to receive feedback and change their own behaviors. Validation is NOT, however, always easy for parents. Often our children will feel or believe things that we know *(or believe, because we're not perfect or all-knowing either)* are either overly simplified, wrongly interpreted, or just plain wrong. The good news is that validating your child doesn't mean you agree with their feelings or actions.

The bad news is that the opposite of validation is so, so easy to do. It's easy and tempting, for instance, to tell your child they shouldn't be depressed because they are so smart, or talented, or that they have so many friends, so many people who care about them. We desperately want our children to see themselves as we see them, and understand how deeply loved they are. We are SO tempted to argue with their feelings, correct them, point out where they are wrong and that things are really not as bad as they are saying. This approach, really, is our own attempt to minimize their pain in order to reduce our own fear and anxiety.

We don't appreciate it as adults when other people tell us that our feelings are wrong, illogical, or silly. *(ESPECIALLY if those other people are married to us, but I digress.)* If you've ever been told to "c'mon, just smile" on a terrible, awful day, or "I just don't see the big deal," about something you think IS a big deal, then you know how your kids feel when it's done to them.

Rather, we should practice so that we can listen intently and without judgment. Ask open-ended questions that cannot be answered with a simple yes or no. Resist the urge to offer quick fixes or solutions to their challenges, which tends to shut down further dialogue.

Listen, and then ask, "this is what I'm hearing. Did I get it right?" Follow their cues, and then say things like:

- "Tell me more about that. I'd love to understand more about what that's like for you."

- "I'm sorry you are feeling so bad. I want to help."

- "It feels really bad now but it's not always going to feel this way. How can we help you get through this crisis?"

- "Hey, I've noticed you've been really quiet lately, is everything okay?" (Or really irritable, or sad, or whatever you've noticed.)

- "You are so strong, and I'm so proud of you for talking about this/for going to therapy/for working so hard when you feel so bad."

Note: using the word strong with your child is important. They probably do not see themselves as strong, but they are, simply for what they've already achieved. Living with depression, or OCD, or other serious mental illnesses, or trauma, is brutally difficult. Helping them see their own strength is helping them build the resilience they need to grow even stronger. Use the word strong.

Try not to be overly shocked by your child's words or behaviors. Your child is experiencing intense emotions without the coping skills to manage them, and what they say is merely their momentary expression of those intense, overwhelming feelings through the prism of that lack of coping. They are having emotions they cannot handle and their behavior is the best they can do right now. If they could do better, they would do better. *(If that statement annoys you, if you argue with it, if you don't believe that about your child, you may be like me. You may have been raised in a model that said, "Oh, HELL NO, if they WANTED to do better, they would do better." If that resonates with your internal wrestling, I HIGHLY recommend you Google Dr. Ross Green and "kids do well if they can." It's not easy for some of us to accept, depending on how we were raised, but it will change everything about the way you approach the struggles your child has.)*

In other words, if they say they hate everything and they will never ever want to live, try to hear that as an expression not of truth, but of depression and hopelessness. ***Remember, that is not your child's truth talking, it is their depression talking.*** Not only that, but it is their depression talking RIGHT NOW IN THIS MOMENT.

Those thoughts and fears are not necessarily true just because they are feeling that way right now. The problem, of course, is that we don't always know when our brains are lying to us, especially when we are struggling with mental illness. It's when we believe those feelings that we can be in danger, and can contemplate or act on suicidal feelings. We can help our children learn that depression and anxiety will lie to them, and just because our brain feels something doesn't always make it true.

I do not usually swear in front of my children, but for what it's worth I have found in parenting that the occasional, well-placed curse word can be effective. This is why I recently told my child that her depression is a total asshole. I want to help her externalize her depression. It is not her truest self, no matter what it tells her, and despite the fact her depression will tell her just about anything to protect itself.

What if they don't want to talk?

If they don't want to talk, leave the invitation open. Make sure they know that you are here for them when they're ready; that you will listen and support them; and that you won't judge them, no matter what they're going through.

Also, just because they don't want to talk doesn't mean they can choose not to listen if there are important facts, issues or thoughts you want to share. *(Especially if you limit your sharing judiciously, says a mom with a tendency to go on and on.)* They may roll their eyes, they may appear not to be listening, but some of what you say will sink in. I mean, that's parenting, right? I'm just reiterating that here because when we are parenting suicidal kids, we can forget to continue operating on basic parenting modes such as "Talk Even If It Looks Like They Are Ignoring You," which are still entirely valid and appropriate.

My daughter is a private, internal processor who keeps things pretty close to the vest, in general. This has been hard for me, as a VERY externally processing person. Sometimes it feels like she doesn't even want to tell me what she had for lunch let alone dissect the current status of her mental health, which of course I would LOVE to do.

The solution? I've had to learn to give her space, to back off, to respect the fact that this is HER journey and not mine. She owes a tremendous debt of gratitude to her older cousin, K, because these were all lessons that I had to learn and practice with K first, and I can promise you they did NOT come easy to me. They still don't, if I'm being honest, but I'm getting better.

Now that we are not in immediate crisis territory *(I believe. I think. Just being real.)* I've found that if I really need to talk with A, it helps to give her advance notice instead of just popping into her bedroom unannounced or snagging her attention when she comes out for snacks. How did I come to know that strategy worked better? When she said, "Mom, it stresses me out and is unhelpful when you pop into my bedroom unannounced *(I mean, I DO knock)* or pounce on me when I come out for snacks."

I'm a quick learner. *(No, I'm not.)* *(She is learning boundaries and self-advocacy in therapy, yay!)*

We still have days or weeks when my mom senses begin to tingle, or when I am seeing red flags (usually increased isolation or irritability), and I am concerned about her and feel the need to check in with her, or sometimes I just need to check in on therapy or other things. So I will either text her and tell her I'd like to touch base and talk, or mention it when she comes out for snacks, and ask her to make time for me that day. This seems to work, as she has time to think about it, prepare, and not feel ambushed.

By the way, my mom senses are usually spot on, and I've found that when those alarm bells begin to ring, I've been right that she's struggling. We plan to check in, and she's been willing to share what's up, if she needs anything, and if we can help. Sometimes we can, more often there isn't anything we can do except know she's struggling and be a bit more watchful. My point in sharing that? You know your kid. Trust your gut, and carefully but directly check in with them if you're worried.

Obviously, when immediate safety is at question, you can't accept zero communication, and you will have to work with your child to establish a bare minimum check-in strategy that allows them their space and privacy but gives you the information you need to help keep them safe. If they won't communicate at all, they need to understand that then you will be operating on incomplete information and might not be able to help in a way they would want, AND that you have some fair, basic expectations that they need to work toward meeting.

The likelihood is that your child will open up when you least expect it, sitting side-by-side rather than face-to-face, in the car or engaged in some other activity together. Or, in my experience, they'll be ready and want to talk about 11:30 p.m., late on a night that you had a horrible day at work, the cat barfed all over the living room, and you had to rewash the laundry because you forgot to start the dryer three days ago.

Ah, parenting. But if they want to talk, we talk!

What not to say

Here are some approaches to talking with your suicidal child that are unlikely to help. I've gathered these anti-suggestions from experts, and also from my own mistakes and experience. Some of them may feel like exactly the RIGHT or natural thing to say, but hear me out.

As I have learned from people who have been suicidal, in those moments they aren't trying to hurt anyone, and they are not trying to get attention. Sure, their mental illness may be telling them lies like "your family would be better off without you" or "there is no point in trying anymore, it won't get any better," but you cannot argue with an irrational mind that is struggling with mental illness. You will not be able to reason anyone out of their suicidal feelings.

You will not be able to reason anyone out of their suicidal feelings.

Not only that but in the worst moments, they literally cannot factor in how their actions would affect you or anyone else, because they JUST WANT THE PAIN TO STOP. They want the pain they are feeling, the depression, or the hopelessness, to stop. They see no other path forward and no hope for life to get better.

Things we might say that REALLY don't help

"Everything is going to be okay."

It does not feel that way to them, that is not their experience right now, and that tells them you aren't listening or paying attention. This type of statement is invalidating. You know what happens when we invalidate people? They shut down, and they stop sharing honestly with us because they believe (even if that isn't what we mean) that we aren't going to take them seriously.

Is it likely you are right, that everything IS going to be okay? Sure, I can totally confirm you are likely right, and that eventually everything is going to be okay. See what I did there? I VALIDATED you and your thinking. It feels way better than me telling you "Well, we don't really know if it will be okay, no one knows the future, maybe it won't be." Not only that, but telling them everything is going to be okay is still irrelevant to them in the moment and still unhelpful.

"Do you have any idea how scared I was/how scared I am/how hard this is for me?"

Yeah, this was something I said to K and her therapist a lot, early on, and it was true! The problem is that these types of statements make it all about you. You are the grown up, and this shouldn't be all about you. I was SO offended when K's therapist told me I needed to pull it together because I was making things harder for K, and making it all about me. "How dare she?" I thought. "Does she not realize how difficult this is, how terrified I've been, how this makes me feel . . . oh, yeah, now I see her point."

This parenting journey is nothing if not humbling, that's for sure.

The fact is, when we say things like this to our kids, we put them in the position of having to take care of US, and OUR feelings. Not only does this add to the burden they are already carrying, but it makes them feel like they have to protect us. Even without us doing or saying anything, they have already likely been keeping their feelings in and not sharing openly because they already don't want to upset us, make us sad or scare us.

When our kids feel it is their job to protect US, they share less honestly and openly about their mental health, and that could put them in more danger.

ANYTHING along the lines of "Suicide is a permanent solution to a temporary problem."

They don't need platitudes, bumper stickers or clichés, for crying out loud. Especially not ones that minimize their experiences. It's insulting, and they know it's the easy conversational out. It is rigid, lacking in compassion and honestly disrespectful *(again, even if you don't intend to send that message, doesn't matter.)* Not only that, but this generation of kids is especially sensitive to those types of sayings. They see right through them, and they know there is little there of help.

"But you have so much to live for/you have so many friends/you are so talented . . ."

That is probably true, but it does not feel that way to them, that is not their experience right now, and that tells them you aren't listening or paying attention. This type of statement is invalidating. There will be a time and a place for you to help your child see their own unique, brilliant qualities. In fact that will always be one of your most important jobs as their parent. However, when they are actively in crisis, this just feels like "I'm not really hearing you, what you feel doesn't matter and isn't real." When by definition, what they feel IS real, even when it doesn't make sense to us.

"Do you have any idea of how this would devastate your brother/sister/grandma/dad/mom?"

When your child is in crisis, they are focused on their own pain. They are not being inconsiderate or uncaring of others, they are just consumed by their own overwhelming feelings, and may even feel like others would be better off without them.

"You need to snap out of this and see how good your life really is. You have more than X% of kids on this planet."

Again, that is probably true, but it does not feel that way to them, that is not their experience right now, and that tells them you aren't listening or paying attention. This type of statement is invalidating.

Not only that, but it's a particularly tone-deaf version of the tired parenting trope about cleaning your plate because kids in Africa don't have enough to eat. Let's be real, that never made you want to finish your lima beans when you were a kid, and you weren't even in a mental health crisis!

What do you do if your child refuses to get help?

What if your child is suicidal, or at least lives with regular suicidal thoughts, and you know they need help, but they refuse? They refuse therapy, they don't want to see a psychiatrist, they don't want to go to the emergency room. What do you do?

First, get your own help, ASAP. You will likely need your OWN professional to help guide you through this time, and it should be someone experienced with both adolescents and parents. This is such a difficult situation that you need to source some external ideas, suggestions, and strategies.

Second, begin by thinking about what your child does want, what does motivate them, and how to connect them to getting what they want, with them getting additional help. Think along the lines of, "In our house, we take care of ourselves by getting medical care when we need it, and mental health care IS medical care. I know it's important to you to spend time on YouTube/Instagram/*Fortnite*, and it's important to me that you are getting treatment. So I'm happy to continue to allow you the Wi-Fi password as long as you are making the choice to get treatment/therapy/talk to a doctor."

If your child refuses to see a therapist, try getting them to agree to try three times with a promise (a promise that you WILL honor) that if after those visits, they can't stand it, then they don't have to go back to that person. You may have to try several therapists before your child finds one they feel comfortable with and connects with, but after all, adults go through the same thing. Your child doesn't have to be best friends with their therapists, but they do need to feel comfortable, seen, and heard.

Still facing refusal? Think about who they WILL talk to and accept – is it a baseball coach? Aunt or uncle? Youth group leader? How about the counselor or mental health specialist at school? Even though those important figures in your child's life are NOT mental health providers and should not be expected to be, they can be a lifeline for a child who isn't yet willing to let others in.

If they refuse to go to the emergency room in a crisis

If your child's immediate physical safety is at risk, you may have to be open to calling 911 and involving a community mental health crisis team or even law enforcement. You may have to consider an involuntary hold. The laws for involuntary holds (or commitment) differ from state to state, and with your child's age and your state's legal age of consent to treatment. You will need to look them up. Start researching with the Treatment Advocacy Center, tac.org. If you think it is even a future possibility, do that research now.

Taking such steps will certainly be difficult for you and your child, but if it comes to their safety and they aren't willing to agree to seek help, you may not have any choice. (I say this while acknowledging the reality that any form of involuntary treatment comes with an additional level of potential trauma, and involving law enforcement may bring additional trauma and potential risk to your child, especially for people of color.)

A note on using cell phones as punishment

Maybe . . . don't. I have heard several professionals talk on this subject recently, and their approach surprised me. Certainly, our kids' cell phones are a privilege, and that makes them an easy target for us to remove in the search for appropriate natural consequences. But our kids' cell phones are their primary source of music, connection to their friends, and distraction. And sure, there is probably a perfectly healthy teen who is just choosing to be a brat, or making bad choices, for whom losing their cell phone makes sense.

But natural consequences often aren't an effective approach with kids who are struggling with serious mental health issues. They desperately need connection to their friends and the outside world, and they cannot access the logic and maturity, let alone the emotional bandwidth, necessary to benefit from what seems like a logical natural consequence.

This is a great example of how standard parenting approaches don't work for every kid, and how parenting isn't always going to be fair. Equitable, yes, in that you want each child to receive the support and guide rails that they need to be well and thrive, but not fair, in that different children need different things.

Let me give you an example of how we made this mistake, and what it cost one of our children. Our oldest child was really struggling in high school with completing and turning in homework, and while we sort of suspected he had ADHD, it would be years before he was willing to talk about and consider it as a possibility. Meanwhile, we also suspected that maybe he just wasn't trying hard enough, maybe he was spending too much time playing video games on his computer and his phone, and maybe if we took those away as a consequence for bad grades it would help him pull it together.

I KNOW. I KNOW. That was a terrible idea, and not only did we take away his phone and computer, but we did it for *(*me, cringing in shame*)* months. *(Again, we need to forgive ourselves and give ourselves grace. We do the best we can as parents with what we know. This memory still hurts, however.)*

Did it turn around his academic situation? No, of course not, because effort wasn't his issue, executive function was. What it DID do was nearly completely cut him off from his friends, and the primary way they communicated, and the way they spontaneously planned going out together. We isolated him from a teenager's most important social contacts.

Thank goodness he didn't have major depression, because I can't imagine how that would have impacted him. As I said, I've since heard several mental health professionals state that isolating a teen through taking their cell phone is rarely a good idea.

Not only that, but as discussed, your child's cell phone is probably a key tool in their safety plan tool kit. It can be a way for them to remind themselves of their tools, to access their safety plan, to contact the folks on their safety plan, and reach out for help. In a safety emergency, it can also be a way to track your child's location.

(We did do some things right, however. Our kids' cell phones ALWAYS spent the night in the kitchen, so they weren't distracted by texts from their friends or the temptation of video games when their brains needed the crucial healing and growing that happens during sleep. At least until they were of college age and were able to make their own bad cell phone decisions like we sometimes do.)

Don't make it all about mental health

Talk about other things, too.

It can be easy for your conversations with your child to become heavily focused on their emotional state, their therapy appointments, their prescription refills, safety check-ins, etc. But your child needs to be reminded that they are NOT their mental health problem. They are still the same funny or smart or quirky or athletic or deep-thinking kid they've always been. Maybe you need that same reminder about them yourself.

Make time to talk about anything else that's NOT mental health related. This is healthy, it's distracting, it makes a deposit into your relational bank with your child, and it's stress relieving. Ask questions that don't have yes or no answers, and lean into their interests or hobbies. Yes, that means you might have to listen to them talk about *Fortnite*, or *Dungeons & Dragons*, ballet, Taylor Swift, or soccer.

Some questions to consider *(obviously, don't ask questions that you know might make things worse)*:

- Who are your friends now? What do you do with them?

- Who would you say is your favorite new musician?

- What's the best video you watched on YouTube today? *(Just being realistic, here, folks.)*

- How is that new video game going? *(Still being realistic.)*

- Can you explain *(thing they learned in school that was news to you, or trend or issue related to teens you read about in the news, etc.)* to me?

Planning for, and talking about, recovery

This section is short, but vitally important.

Probably the most important message you can communicate openly to your child is your absolute expectation for their recovery. We must plan for mental health recovery, just as we plan for mental health crises and emergencies. Talk about recovery as if it is a foregone conclusion, a certainty.

One way to help your child hope and plan for recovery is giving them a way to see their improvement. Work with your child and their therapist or provider to determine how and when you'll know that they are improving. Take note of the improvement when you see it, and call it out. *(Without, heaven forbid, making a big deal about it, or too often, because that's a guaranteed recipe for an eye roll. On the other hand, eye rolls can be a sign of improvement too!)* This is especially important when your child feels hopeless, as it will remind both of you that this is temporary, that they will get better, and that recovery is possible.

Recovery is possible, and, in fact, recovery is the expectation for most people who struggle with mental health issues, even suicidal ideation. Our society doesn't talk enough about recovery from mental illness, but it is real and it is possible. Now, I know that this isn't a guarantee, and I can't give you one of those. Nor can I promise you that recovery is going to look like "back to normal before we could have ever contemplated that our child would think about suicide." In fact, normal may not be in the future, but happiness, hope, joy, and meaning can be.

Believe me, I'm no Pollyanna. I have had many days, weeks and even months, especially with K, in which I saw absolutely no reason to hope for my young person. But slowly, often imperceptibly, things will get better. Okay, sometimes they will get better and then get worse again. You know that saying, "it's a marathon, not a sprint?" Well, that is certainly the case in my family *(and as we've established earlier, I don't even like to run.)*

Please let me believe in recovery for you right now, if you can't, until you can believe it for your child, until they can believe it for themselves. I know when there have been attempts, when you are exhausted from hypervigilance, when you believe they will NEVER get better, it's hard to even hope for recovery.

But more than 90% of people who have made a suicide attempt at some point in their life will die of something other than suicide. The vast majority of people who have lived with suicidal thoughts or who have attempted suicide go on to recover.

It is possible. I promise.

Advocate fiercely

At some point in this journey, if you don't already, you may begin to feel like you know nothing. You don't know how to do this, it's too hard, too scary and too complicated, and the stakes are WAY too high. But here's the deal. No therapist, psychiatrist, school counselor, or other expert will ever love your child more than you, and they will never fight harder for your child than you.

That's your job, the job only you can do, the job no one can do better than you: love your child and fight for your child. You are their best advocate, and you are the best person to teach them how to become their OWN best advocate.

YOU are the expert on your kid

Don't forget that you are the expert on your kid. You know what sets them off, or sends them down a spiral, and you know when your alarm bells are going off and you need to pay attention. You also know what times of day may be hardest for them, and what they need when they are feeling fragile.

Or maybe, you don't. I mean, eventually you will. With my niece K, we knew from the beginning that suicide was a risk for her, and that she had a history of suicidal ideation and self-harm. She still could present as if nothing was wrong.

But with my child, we didn't have a lot of signs. Before her crises, A presented well, socialized beautifully, and largely got on with life in a charming, comfortable way that masked the times she saw no point in life, and she had no desire to "be here" any longer, and she was afraid she would always feel this way.

The only signs we had before we knew A was suicidal happened when we were talking about school, and A's inability to do school well despite being highly intelligent. It was only during the conversations about another bad grade or missing assignment that we heard things like "I just can't do this anymore, it feels hopeless, I just don't care."

In our particular case, it took us WAY too long to find out A also has ADHD in addition to depression and anxiety. *(A very common triumvirate of diagnoses, we've since found out.)* Knowing about the ADHD allowed us to strike on that front as well, although finding effective treatments she can tolerate has been just about as difficult as finding effective treatments for depression and anxiety.

My point is that sometimes even the best parent, the most dialed-in parent, misses the signs. *(I am a professional mental health speaker and I didn't know my own kid had ADHD for more than 17 years! P.S., she was 20 before she was diagnosed with autism.) (I'm definitely not claiming I'm the best or most dialed-in parent, and I get it.)* Some kids either don't have the words for what they are feeling, don't know that their feelings aren't "normal," or they hide their feelings completely. You can't act on, or help with, what you don't know.

Get your facts ready, document everything!

Being an effective advocate for your child requires that you collect accurate data, and that you can tell a complete, concise and compelling story about their experiences to the experts with whom you'll be working.

Document what you know and what you have seen of your child's symptoms. Definitely document specific events and behaviors, but more big picture documentation can also be helpful.

Questions to ask yourself:

- What exactly does their day look like?

- What are the areas of life in which they struggle? Is it school, is it with friends, is it with family?

- How has that changed?

- What have they stopped doing that they used to enjoy? How are they different?

- What symptoms have you observed, or do they report?

- How are their symptoms or behaviors interfering with their ability to function?

- What have you tried, both at home, at school and with other providers?

- What treatment has your child received in the past, what therapies?

- What has worked, what didn't work, what worked but then stopped working?

Be open with providers about any recreational drug use and do your best to let go of judgment with your child when it comes to their drug use so that they will be open with you. The truth is that about 40% percent of our teens and young adults report having used cannabis in the last year, and use of other drugs such as hallucinogens continues to rise. Use of these drugs can significantly impact depression, anxiety and suicidal thinking and their treatment, and their medical team **needs** that information. Use of cannabis is also linked to psychosis and to the onset of schizophrenia, and so it's important that everyone has full information so they can best evaluate and treat your child.

All of this documentation will serve two purposes in getting your child the best treatment:

- First, it will give their provider specific actionable information that can help them pinpoint a diagnosis and the severity of the situation, as well as give them a better understanding of your child as a person.

- Second, documentation will make clear to the provider that you as a parent are organized, informed, in touch, and, therefore, someone to whom they should absolutely pay attention. This second point shouldn't be necessary, but mental health providers are human, and they walk into a treatment room with their own biases or prejudices based on other kids and families. Being able to present your observations efficiently can help cut to the chase and establish the best plan as quickly as possible.

Trust yourself, *and* know you will screw up

Be open-minded when it comes to treatment. Do your research, but stick to the experts, and NOT the ones you find on Instagram. Now isn't the time to humor your Aunt Jane and start your child on a diet of foods that start with i or that contain only ingredients grown in Uzbekistan. It's just not, not when your child's life is at stake. Can you add supplemental, alternative approaches? Sure, absolutely. *(If you are using supplements or dietary approaches, definitely share that information with your traditional providers.)* Nor is it the time to listen to that guy from church who thinks taking medicine is a sin, or makes you weak, or whatever. Now is the time to find experts you trust and follow their lead—with lots of questions and your own knowledge of your child's situation, of course.

You are going to have moment after moment in which you have to look your kid in the eye and make a judgment call. It's okay. You have to do it, and you CAN do it.

What do I do if I can't find a therapist or a psychiatrist?

What can I do if the first available appointment isn't available for three to four months?

Where else can I find help?

Be persistent, and embrace your new role as the polite, delightful, but impossible-to-avoid squeaky wheel.

Keep calling. Don't give up. I know it is disheartening to call 30 therapists or psychiatrists when 12 never called back, 15 don't take your insurance and three have a waiting list. But don't give up. Be polite but be persistent. Ask to be placed on the cancellation list. Tell them you are very flexible and can fill any open appointments. Keep calling. Emphasize that your child has experienced suicidal thinking.

Ask friends for recommendations of providers they've seen *(and liked, ideally, but you gotta start somewhere)*.

Ask your insurance company to help you find a provider. Some insurance companies have case managers or a person in an equivalent position, whose job it is to coordinate more serious cases. Asking for someone like a case manager can get you better connected with the help and resources you need.

Call your local NAMI chapter and ask if they can help. Even if they don't know of providers with openings, they may have classes or support groups for you or your child that would be helpful. NAMI stands for the National Alliance on Mental Illness, and they are a national nonprofit with regional chapters that offer all kinds of evidence-based, FREE support groups; educational classes for parents, caregivers and family members and also for people living with mental illness; and local support lines staffed with people who know local resources and programs.

It was FIVE years before anyone told us about NAMI when we were raising my nieces, and it would have been so helpful if we had known about them earlier.

Surround yourself AND your child with support from your community. Don't be shy. Ask for help from your friends and family, just to be with you and be there for you and your child. Loneliness and isolation are a risk for both of you, and community is healing.

Focus on getting your child connected with activities that encourage their interests. If there is some activity or interest that your child is willing to engage in, now is the time to spend some extra effort, time, and even money if you can. Remember that help and healing is a holistic activity. Helping your child find what they love to do and supporting them in their hobbies and interests can also be a powerful type of therapy.

Use the school. Take advantage of every resource through your child's school. Talk to the school counselor or mental health specialist and let them know you're having a hard time getting your child treatment. They may have resources or connections to providers in your area, and they may be able to make phone calls or even pull strings for you. They can definitely set up regular, even daily check-ins with your child, and establish their office or hallway as a spot for your child to take space when they are overwhelmed or need a break. Establishing one or two people at school with whom your child connects can be a strong protective factor. Research indicates kids who feel connected at school do better with mental health, just like kids who feel connected at home.

Explore area support groups for both you and your child. Support groups can be powerful avenues of healing and may be more accessible than an appointment with a psychiatrist. Google is your friend here.

HIPAA—it doesn't go two ways!

Sometimes when you are working with a provider, a hospital or other facility, and trying to talk with them about your child, you will hear about HIPAA, which is the Health Insurance Portability and Accountability Act. This is a national law (in the U.S.) that, among other purposes, is intended to create systems and policies to prevent the medical and insurance systems from sharing sensitive personal patient data without the patient's (or parents', in the case of a child) permission. However, sometimes that law gets used as an excuse to avoid sharing with parents or other family members, as a way of avoiding liability.

But here's the deal.

You can tell a doctor or nurse anything you want, and you can ask them to listen and take notes. They may not respond with specifics, to protect their patient's privacy, and they may not be allowed to give you information from the patient's medical records if you aren't designated to receive it. Respect their limitations AND tell them they will continue to hear from you. Also, be sure and tell them you appreciate everything that they are doing to help your child and you. *(Remember, you are a delightful squeaky wheel.)*

Laws on this for children, and the ages at which that information is protected, vary from state to state. If your state allows doctors to keep a child or teen's medical information confidential, then, in a CALM moment, encourage your child to sign a release of information form (ROI) with their providers so the providers can speak to you about your child's condition and treatment.

But even without a signed ROI, a therapist or a doctor can listen to you, take in what you are sharing, and hopefully factor it into their approach with your child. They may not be able to respond, or give you ANY information in return, but they can listen. There is NO rule against that, and listening is NOT a HIPAA violation.

Listening to you is NOT a HIPAA violation. In fact, to provide good patient care, they have a responsibility to listen to you.

This will be even more important for you to keep in mind if your child lives with serious mental health issues into adulthood.

Not only that, but providers can ALWAYS give you general information. You can ask: What types of general guidance do you give in a situation in which a child is suicidal, or a child is self-harming, or whatever you are experiencing with your kid? They can always give you general, nonspecific guidance.

Of course, remember that it is absolutely important that your child has a confidential relationship with their providers that they can trust. Their therapist will never and should never tell you what your child is saying without your child's permission. But with a release of information or your child's permission, it can be reasonable and helpful for the therapist or doctor to share general information on a treatment plan, ways you can support your child at home, things you may be doing that are NOT supportive of your child, and of course medication changes.

Working with the school

If your child is suicidal, you need to talk with the school. They need to know what's going on so they can support your child and help keep them safe. Start with the school mental health specialist or counselor, or the teacher, but start the conversation.

Ideally, when you share your child's mental health situation with their school, the school will lean in and be willing to get equipped if they aren't already. The school should respond out of skill and empathy, and not out of fear of liability. This may sound obvious, but I call it out because there is a chance that may NOT be the situation you face, either at a system level or at an individual level with teachers.

Just like every other facet of society, teachers may face their own internalized stigma surrounding mental health. Schools have begun doing a much better job educating teachers and others in the school system about mental health and about suicide prevention, but that doesn't guarantee the messages have sunk in with everyone.

If an education professional *(or any trusted adult)* approaches a mental health situation with judgment, students may feel invalidated and replicate this stigma in their own lives. In contrast, if a teacher approaches mental health topics with compassion and empathy, they create a healthier culture in which students will ask for the help they need.

If you get even a HINT that a teacher or other education professional is sharing judgmental, ignorant, or unhelpful messages with your child, you should jump on that immediately. Start with the teacher and give them a chance to do better, but if that doesn't happen quickly, escalate as far up as you need to go to get action and cooperation to protect your child. *(Remember, your role is polite, persistent, and delightful squeaky wheel.)*

The good news is that schools are better equipped now than ever before to help kids who are struggling with mental health. There is more focus, more training and more resources. Unlike when we were in school, many schools now have mental health specialists *(often licensed therapists)* in addition to school counselors, and they can be a tremendous resource for your child and for you. They can work with your child's teacher or teachers to develop strategies to help your child stay engaged, feel safe, and have reasonable accommodations.

I say reasonable accommodations because mental illness is a protected disability. Mental illness, or emotional disturbance in school lingo (an unfortunate phrase but that's the term used by the government), may qualify your child for additional help and resources through special education. Don't get weird about the term "special ed." What's most important is that this is simply an extra way to possibly get help for your child. Even if your child is a straight "A" student who before now has never needed any help at school, this is simply the department through which help for kids with mental health issues is funneled. It might mean an ongoing plan for support like a 504 plan or an Individualized Education Program (IEP.) It's okay if you don't know what those are; now is a great time to head to the resources in the back of this book and start learning!

Public schools (and universities and some private schools with limitations) are obligated to conduct an individual assessment of any student believed to need special education or related services because of a disability, in order to provide the student with a free appropriate public education. Know your child's rights as you advocate for them with the school.

"I told the school, but I'm not getting any help."

- Who did you tell? Was it the right people? Keep trying!
- What are they going to do with your information? Ask for follow-up steps!
- What do you WANT them to do with that info? Have a goal in mind going into every conversation about what your ideal outcome for your child is.
- Did you teach them how to support your kid? Should you have to? No, but sometimes that's your job too.

One expert with whom I spoke had a cool suggestion. Create a one-page document that you can provide to the school that includes three things that help your child or make their experience better, and three things that you know make things worse for your child. This could also be provided to youth group leaders, coaches, Scout leaders, etc.

Don't worry about credits, grades, etc.

I remember one of K's early IEP meetings, a big team meeting with her school counselor, therapist, caseworker, teachers, an administrator, and even her insurance care coordinator. K was fresh out of her latest hospitalization for suicidal ideation, and yet there I was, verbally agonizing over why no one seemed concerned that K's class assignments were not optimized to make her ready and attractive to colleges.

Everyone around the table, heck, including K, just . . . stared at me. They were focused on how to keep her safe since much of each school day involved K getting triggered, bolting, disassociating, and hiding in the bathroom to self-harm. Meanwhile, I was fretting about whether we had the ideal selection of college prep classes?!?

I'm sure they all spent a lot of those meetings internally shaking their heads and thinking, "Bless her heart . . ." But like all parents of kids who live with mental illness, I had to learn completely new expectations and completely new ways to parent that are not covered in the standard parenting directions that come with the baby. *(Or the foster niece.) (Oh, wait . . . standard parenting directions aren't even a thing.)*

Accept, love and support your LGBTQ kid

If your child falls into the LGBTQ community, ***find a way to be supportive and accepting***. I'm not going to dance around this or give you any kind of an out.

It may save your child's life.

The discrimination and rejection that LGBTQ kids anticipate and frequently receive from the world is crushing. Bullying is still rampant for these kids, and the sociopolitical landscape is filled with trauma, discrimination, hate, and misinformation. This is the world in which they are growing up, and this world is dangerous for their mental health. *(By the way, our BIPOC kids are at similar increased risk because of discrimination.)*

Kids who report that their families, their school, and their community are not accepting or supportive of their gender identity or sexual orientation are at higher risk of attempting suicide, and dying by suicide. That is a fact.

According to thousands of respondents to the 2022 National Survey on LGBTQ Youth Mental Health by the Trevor Project:

- **LGBTQ youth who report having at least one accepting adult were 40% less likely to report a suicide attempt in the past year.**

- LGBTQ youth from families that are highly rejecting are EIGHT TIMES more likely to attempt suicide.

- LGBTQ youth who felt high social support from their family reported attempting suicide at less than half the rate of those who felt low or moderate social support.

- Nearly 20% of LGBTQ teens attempted to die by suicide in the past year.

If you live in a state or a part of the country that is trying to pass anti-LGBTQ legislation, you need to know that your kid is paying attention, and it matters. In states where such legislation is proposed, research has found a significant rise in the rates of kids contacting crisis hotlines. Research by the Trevor Project found a shocking 72% increase in suicide attempts among trans and nonbinary youth in states that have recently passed anti-trans laws. You read that right, a 72% increase in suicide attempts.

Our kids are watching, and the words and actions of politicians, lawmakers, and religious leaders can be dangerous to our kids, who often feel like they are living in a world that wants to deny their existence.

And having just one adult who accepts them for who they are is highly protective. Whether they are gay, transgender, bisexual, or gender fluid, whatever, **it doesn't matter if you don't get it**, or if you don't understand. It doesn't matter whether you believe that your child is walking into their true identity as whom they were created to be, or whether you think they are making a lifestyle choice or responding to a trend *(this latter belief is not borne out in the data, btw)*.

If they want you to use different pronouns or a different name, for the love of your child, do it.

THIS IS THEIR TRUE EXPERIENCE RIGHT NOW IN THIS MOMENT. Your response, and your support, as their parent or guardian means everything.

Love them. Support them. That is your job. If you are not willing to do that job, it may cost you your child's life.

It is as simple as that.

What about cutting and self-harm?

Finding out that your child has been intentionally hurting themselves by cutting, scratching or burning themselves can be horrifying. Until K first came to live with us and her caseworker told us that she often cut herself, I had never even heard of cutting. It also makes you wonder about their safety and wonder if it means your child is actively suicidal, and, in fact, many kids who have struggled with self-harm have also struggled with suicidal thoughts.

Cutting, or other types of self-injury, is not necessarily a sign of someone who is actively suicidal, and most of the time cutting and self-harm episodes are not suicide attempts. Cutting IS a sign of deep emotional distress that requires treatment, and, when ignored, that distress could deepen and become suicidal thinking.

Cutting is viewed as an attempt to either generate sensation that seeks to distract from overwhelming, painful emotions; interrupt those seemingly intolerable emotions; or to generate any sensation when a person is feeling hopeless, numb, and disconnected from themselves. In other words, people self-harm to help them not feel feelings that seem impossible to tolerate, or to feel any other feelings than those intolerable emotions.

Obviously, young people are impulsive and self-harm can go wrong; it needs to be taken very seriously. Self-injury can result in scarring, infection, and other medical complications.

But like suicidal behaviors, self-harm is also a behavior, a maladaptive behavior to an experience your child doesn't yet have the tools to handle in a healthy way. Self-harm can also be self-reinforcing because of the chemicals it releases in the brain that do in fact provide a sense of temporary relief. Thus, it can become a compulsive behavior that is difficult to stop, so early action and treatment is necessary.

Treatment involves a lot of skill building, so that their tool bucket is full and equipped with other options when they are struggling. They may need to develop tolerance of uncomfortable or painful emotions, radical acceptance of difficult situations, healthy ways of distraction, and methods of grounding themselves in the present moment.

Three pieces of good news about these types of skills:

1. These skills are also useful in overcoming suicidal ideation. Again, self-harm and suicidal ideation aren't the same, but some of the same skills and tools can be helpful in healing both.

2. These skills are ALL very useful for parents of teens and children struggling with mental illness. Learning them and PRACTICING them with your child is a win-win for everyone!

3. These skills are actually universally useful for all humans, and learning them will make your child stronger for their entire life journey.

Cutting and other forms of self-harm is also a good opportunity to practice another important parenting skill—NOT FREAKING OUT.

When my niece was self-harming, we were taught to react calmly, in a practical manner, and without huge amounts of dramatic compassion.

I know this is far easier said than done. Finding out that your child is literally injuring themselves can be shocking, scary, confusing, and can even cause us feelings of disgust or anger.

Not freaking out accomplishes two important goals: it prevents any possible maladaptive attention-seeking increase in the behavior, and it continues to support communication between you and your child so they are comfortable being honest and open with you. Overly emotional responses shut our kids down. *(Believe me, I know that isn't easy. I am a frequent, serious competitor for the crown of Queen of Overly Emotional.)*

Whenever we became aware of a new injury, we checked it out ourselves to make sure medical attention wasn't required, and if it was, we arranged that. If it wasn't required, we made sure that K had the appropriate first aid supplies and training she needed to keep the injury or wound clean and dry to prevent infection, and made it clear we expected her to do just that. (Obviously, this will vary depending on the child, their age, their ability to handle such basic first aid care, and the instructions of their medical team.)

We were told by her treatment team to calmly respond that we were sorry she was feeling that way, and it was a bummer that she had chosen that action to handle those feelings. Sometimes, we did a little review of other ways she could have used her tools, and sometimes we left that for a discussion with the therapist.

We have been with the same pediatrician for our entire parenting journey, and he became K's primary doctor when she came to live with us. I will probably never be more grateful to him than I was when I had to bring K in for treatment of a serious burn she'd given herself with a cigarette lighter. *(That happened when I forgot to check the socks I'd packed for her carefully enough when she was admitted for one of her many hospitalizations, as referenced earlier. We parents are going to miss things, even with the best intentions and information.)*

He was so calm, nonjudgmental, and kind with K. There was no horror, no shaming, no overly dramatic sympathy, just a mellow assessment and rebandaging, with instructions for at-home care.

A note on marijuana

Marijuana is now legal in more states than it is illegal. For consenting adults who have fully formed frontal lobes and the ability to make their own informed decisions, that's fine.

But for our kids, it's been a disaster. Our emergency rooms are full of young people who are experiencing psychosis, severe anxiety, and suicidal depression because they think it is completely safe to use cannabis, because if it wasn't, it wouldn't be legal, right? Wrong. I credit so much of what I have learned about the dangers of marijuana to our kids and their mental health to my friend Julie A. Fast, author and brain health expert on the topics of bipolar, schizoaffective disorder, depression, anxiety, and psychosis. (For more on Julie's books, see Additional Resources.)

As adults, we haven't been in front of this issue because, as Julie says, too many of us think that the marijuana on the streets today is the same weed that Cheech and Chong were enjoying, and it's NOT. *(Don't know who Cheech and Chong are? They were two actors who made comedic movies in the late 70's and early 80's involving titles like "Up in Smoke" and "Still Smokin'." Yes, I'm old. No, I've never actually seen a Cheech and Chong movie.)*

In fact, the marijuana available on the streets today is far stronger than anything available in the 70's, 80's or even 90's.

Kids who use marijuana are seven times more likely to experience psychosis, and there is evidence that marijuana use can drastically worsen mental health issues including depression, anxiety, and bipolar disorder. There is also some evidence that once a mental health issue has been exacerbated, that might create a new baseline of severity.

There are now so many ways that kids can use cannabis, and many of them are very easy to hide. Not only that, but many adults now openly have and use cannabis products in their home without realizing the danger to which they may be exposing their kids.

Does that sound ridiculously alarmist? Am I just a throwback to the days of "just say no to drugs?" No. I'm not. I just want you to be fully informed, so you can have calm, informed discussions with your child and help them make the best possible decisions for their health. OR, assuming that train has left the station, you can be aware of and educated about the possible way cannabis is influencing your child's mental health.

What will people think?

What about the neighbors? What will your mother-in-law say? What about your own parents, or all of your friends?

You don't have time or energy to care. So, don't.

You are now on a parenting journey you didn't choose and for which you didn't prepare. Consequently, you may sometimes feel isolated or lonely due to the different obstacles you and your child are facing, and the different milestones you are trying to reach as a parent of a child with serious mental illness. The truth is that you will find yourself making decisions other parents won't understand and may struggle to support.

You will need to stand strong in your convictions; trust the process that you, your child, and their team developed; and be willing to be misunderstood when necessary. That's okay. Other parents don't know because they haven't been where you are. *(Except that there are SO MANY more parents who have faced this than you even know. We just do a terrible job of talking and connecting with each other about mental illness and suicide.)*

Don't I Could Never

When I speak to general audiences, I often tell them not to "I could never" anyone:

"I could never put my child on medication."

"I could never take them to the ER for a psych evaluation."

"I could NEVER send my child away."

"I could never admit them to the hospital psych unit, or residential mental health treatment."

If you are facing or have faced any of those choices, and someone has "I could never'd" you, it's made your decision more difficult with shame and judgement attached. I'm sorry.

AND, maybe, you have even done that to yourself. You may be self-inflicting your own spirit with thoughts like:

"What kind of parent am I?"

"I'm a terrible parent if I put my child on medication."

"I'm a terrible parent if I take them to the ER for a psych evaluation."

"I'm a terrible parent if I admit them to the hospital psych unit, or residential mental health treatment."

STOP.

Sometimes the best thing we can possibly do for our child is to yield them to specialists who can reach them when we can't. Sometimes that is the difference between a child who gets better and a child who continues to be miserable. Sometimes, that is the difference between life and death.

All of the time, doing these impossibly hard things for your child is the strongest, bravest parenting you can do.

If you receive those types of statements from friends or family? Or if those are your own thoughts? Well . . . the best response is ***I ain't got time for that***.

· · · · · · ·

In fact, I need you to imagine a wall around you, your family, and your child. There is a gate in that wall, and YOU are in charge of who comes through that gate. If there are people in your life who do not understand your child's experience, your experience, or the decisions you are making for your child's health, and they are unsupportive, unkind, critical or otherwise lacking in compassion and respect, you get to decide if the gate opens to them. Those people might be friends, folks at church, or even your parents. It doesn't matter who they are. If they show no signs of attempting to learn more, understand better, or at a minimum respecting and accepting that you are the parent and you are doing your darnedest to do the best for your child, that gate needs to be locked to those people, at least for now.

Before minimizing contact, and IF you have the energy, you can try to offer some education, or just send them some websites to read. You can establish some firm boundaries about what conversation is not helpful or supportive. I.e., "Mom, when you continue to bring up these alternative medicines, or go on and on about medication side effects, you're not helping. You're making all of this harder. I need you to trust my parenting and the team we've put together for our child, or I'm not going to be able to talk to you as much for a while."

It is not selfish to minimize contact with people who make you second guess yourself, or make constant unhelpful suggestions about how you should treat your child's major depressive disorder with more prayer and the essential oils; or how you should just tell your kid to shape up and stop being an entitled snowflake; and who will not listen and respect what YOU need.

Nope, you ain't got time for that. Buh-bye. Imaginary gate in your imaginary family fence locked, you've got things to do. That's not selfish. It's good parenting, it's self-preservation, and it's okay. EVEN if they mean well. EVEN if they are family. EVEN if they are your parents. It's okay.

This is why it is so important to surround yourself with people who either DO get it or who are willing to support you even if they don't get it. You will need to have your own solid support system to withstand the challenges, and they will still be hard. If you don't already have at least one or two close friends or family members with whom you can share, be bold and start seeking them out now. You need them.

A note about faith communities

I hope that if you are a member of a faith community, as I am, that you find comfort and peace there, and you and your family are loved. I also hope that faith community is supportive and open about mental health. Too many faith traditions still have an unspoken taboo about mental health, mental illness, and suicide. Too many churches, for instance, still communicate unhelpful or even harmful messages about mental illness and suicide, continuing to define mental illness as a lack of prayer, a result of sin, or a character defect.

Some faith traditions do not have a history of discussing mental health, and instead will couch mental health issues as spiritual issues.

I happen to be a Christian, and, in my view, mental illness, like any physical illness, is a normal part of the human experience in a broken world. My faith tradition, and my faith community, supports that view and has provided me with tremendous support and comfort over the years. They have made it comfortable and safe for us to share our family's struggles, to be loved without judgment, and to know others are praying for us.

But I also know that I'm lucky.

When I produce conferences for faith communities on mental health, I always hear heartbreaking stories about ways in which churches have made families feel isolated, ashamed, alone, and unloved by God and by the church. It's wrong, and it needs to change.

For the purposes of this book, just know this. If you are a person of faith but in a faith tradition or community that does not have an open, positive, and supportive attitude about mental health, FIND ANOTHER FAITH COMMUNITY. If you are not in crisis now but you are struggling, and your faith community is not supportive, FIND ANOTHER FAITH COMMUNITY.

Someday, when things are calm and smooth, you will have the luxury, if you want, of working with and teaching a faith community to help them learn, grow, and do better. But it is likely that if you are reading this book, you ain't got time for that. Not now.

You need support from all relevant sides, and if faith is important to you, find a community ASAP that will welcome you and your child, and love you through a mental health crisis without shame or judgment.

When to share

When do you share what is happening with your suicidal child? When and as you are able, you can share what is going on in a way that is supportive of and agreeable to you and your child.

It is frankly stupid that we don't talk more openly about mental health issues, and I PROMISE you that when you do share what is happening in your family and with your child, you will be shocked at how many people will immediately, in return, share their mental health struggles and journey.

When you are able to share your family's experiences, it will help reduce the ongoing stigma of mental health issues, and it will also bring you unexpected sources of support.

Honest. It's no different than when you were absolutely sure that your child was the only kid who bit the other kids in kindergarten, or was the only three-year-old who wasn't potty trained. There are so many families going through the same struggles as you or who have gone through those struggles in the past.

Not only that, but you and your child have nothing to be ashamed of, because it is not shameful to experience mental health problems. It is not because you or your child didn't try hard enough, or because you need to change their diet, or because you aren't praying enough, or because you let them have a cell phone too early. *(Sure, the cell phone and every other screen in their life may be contributing to the overall situation, but that's true of every family—and frankly every person—in the developed world. So, you don't have time or energy to deal with that either!)*

Remember, mental health is physical health, and mental health problems are a common part of the human experience. You may feel like you are all alone, but you are not.

I promise you that when you do choose to share your family's experiences, it will help reduce the ongoing stigma of mental health issues, and will bring you unexpected sources of support.

However, it is also true that it will probably result in people saying unhelpful, even stupid things, because that's what humans do, especially when it comes to a topic that makes us feel awkward, or scared, or about which we have misconceptions. So don't feel like you have to share, or that you have to go into great detail until you are ready and until your child is ready.

Note: remember, especially if your child is older, that their mental health is THEIR story. It is their right to determine how much of it you or your family shares, and with whom. NOT because they should be embarrassed or ashamed about what they are going through, but because respecting them in this way is the right thing to do. Asking for and respecting their permission about their story gives them a good example of how to build the boundaries they will need in life, especially if their mental health struggle may be an ongoing issue.

Ask them FIRST if it is okay to tell Grandma, or your book group, or even their friends, all while being clear that mental health struggles, while private, are NOT shameful or anything to be embarrassed about. Don't be surprised if your child is actually far more comfortable being open than you are. Our kids often experience far less internalized stigma and fewer concerns about mental health than we do, and they may be perfectly comfortable telling their friends exactly what is going on. If they are, it's your job to support that while helping them share appropriately. Work together on what they would like to share and how they would like it to be communicated. If they have missed school or have been in the hospital, they need to be ready to tell people something, but you can help them frame it in a way they feel good about. They need to have some autonomy and some control over this, especially when they may feel like they have very little control over anything else in their life.

However, there is an exception to letting your child have complete say over what is shared. YOU need a few people that you trust with whom you can share. Although this is your child's journey, it is also your journey as a parent, and you need to be able to share your fears, worries, and concerns. Often, your spouse or partner may not be enough, and a couple of really close friends or family members can shoulder the additional weight of walking alongside you. *(Is it a gender stereotype to say this is most often true for women, for moms, who may want and need to talk about it WAY more than their husbands? Yes it is. It is also often true.*

Just ask my husband.) Choose carefully, making sure these are people who will empathize but not overreact, who can control the urge to tell you what to do *(thus your mom is sometimes not the best choice)*, and who will KEEP IT TO THEMSELVES.

In addition to your own close friends, remember that getting your own therapist can also be a key part of your support network. Sometimes what we need can be too much for our friends and family. More on that later.

A word about siblings

If life was a math problem, I'm guessing you would be spending maybe 70% of your time, energy, and emotions on your child with suicidal thoughts right now. Throw in basic survival functioning at work and home (18%?), dealing with all of this with your spouse (10%), and remembering to feed the cat (2%). Sure, you have other kids, but what you're dealing with already adds up to 100%, and they're fine.

Right? They're probably fine. I mean, you do a good job of trying not to talk too much about this in front of them, and sure, they know something is up with their sibling, but they're fine. Right?

I know you don't need one more thing to worry about, and your other kids probably ARE fine. But as you can, when you can, make sure you are checking in with them, asking them if they have any questions, and talking openly with them about their sibling at an age-appropriate level. Remember, this isn't just happening to your child and to you. It's a family emergency and a family illness, affecting your other kids, too, and they will need special care and attention from you during this difficult family time. If you are feeling scared and helpless, it's likely that to some degree your other kids are feeling that way too.

(I know, the time/energy/emotion math as laid out above is already 100%. But we get extra percentages when we become parents, so it is possible to use >100%. Plus, maybe you could just feed the cat twice as much, half as often. Maybe do the same with your spouse.)

RESPONSES TO UNHELPFUL SUGGESTIONS OR TIPS THAT SOMEONE'S UNCLE LARRY FOUND ON THE INTERNET

If *(OK, let's be honest, **when**)* people do say stupid things, I have found that having a few pat responses at the ready reduces the energy and emotions I expend on the response, while reducing the effect the comments have on me.

- "Thanks, but we've got a great medical team we trust, and we are closely following their guidance."

- "Hmmm . . . interesting. Thanks for sharing."

- "Oh, gosh, I really appreciate your concern."

- "Are you freaking kidding me? That is not helpful, kind or even accurate. Stop talking." *OK, don't use that one except in really egregious circumstances, when really stupid harmful things are said, especially in your child's presence. Our kids need to know we have their back. But I also just wanted to give you mental permission to at least think it while smiling and nodding as Aunt Gertrude tells you that back in her day, they would have told these kids to just get over it. Geez, Aunt Gertrude.*

Our kids usually realize when something is going on, but if they don't understand it, or the situation is shrouded in secrecy, then they will likely make up explanations that may be far worse than reality. Not only that, but secrecy makes kids feel insecure, and the confusion and worry from having a sibling struggling with their mental health can lead the other kids to develop poor coping strategies, or even higher rates of depression and anxiety.

Watch your other kids for signs of depression and anxiety, including the physical symptoms that can be more common for kids, such as stomachaches and headaches, intense worry, and sleep problems.

Talk about other adults in their life who they would feel comfortable reaching out to for help, and if you feel that they are struggling, don't hesitate to get them their own therapist. Raising families takes a village, and in the case of a family struggling with a family member's mental health, it can take a village PLUS a coach, a youth group leader, a teacher, aunt, uncle, AND a therapist.

You may also be able to find a support group for siblings of kids with mental health issues, which could provide them an opportunity to share and hear from peers in the same situation.

Just as it isn't easy to parent a child with mental health issues—particularly suicidality—it isn't easy to be their brother or sister, either. Siblings can experience many of the same feelings we parents do, without the maturity to process the situation or those feelings in the same way.

Siblings often experience:

- Confusion about behaviors and outbursts from sibling.
- Feeling like they have to walk on eggshells.
- Fear for their sibling's safety.
- Resentment over the amount of attention the sibling is receiving.
- Shame or embarrassment.
- Parentification— taking on adult care-taking behaviors too early.

- Increased independence and resourcefulness.
- Avoidance.
- Anger and resentment—none of this is fair for anybody!
- Increased emotional intelligence.
- Hesitation to burden their parents with their problems, because their parents are already worried or scared for the suicidal sibling.

Tips for helping the siblings of your child with a mental health issue:
- Talk openly and honestly, in an age-appropriate way.
- Give siblings talking points and help them know what to say to friends, family, and school.
- Validate their feelings; let them know that you hear them.
- Spend one-on-one time with them.
- Help them identify other caring adults they can reach out to, especially in an emergency.
- Practice good self-care so you aren't always on empty for your other children.
- Connect with other parents.
- Model healthy relationships.

Recognize that siblings of children who struggle with mental health issues such as depression, anxiety, or suicidal ideation are at increased risk themselves. Make sure that your other kids know that they should talk to you if they begin to experience mental health issues. Because they are probably already worried about you as well as their sibling, reassure them that although you are worried about and helping their sibling, that of course you absolutely have the capacity to be there for them too. *(Do you actually have additional capacity? Who knows? Probably not. But fake it and then get more help.)*

If you have been reading all of this with a sinking feeling in your gut, that was not my intention. Especially since that's how I felt just researching this. "Great, one more way I'm failing as a parent." It's okay. You're doing the best you can with the information, time, and resources you have, just like I am. Consider this a reminder to check in with the other kids in the family, spend some one-on-one time with them, and continue contributing to funds for them to get therapy too someday. *(Kidding. Not kidding.)*

Not Optional:
Take Care of Yourself

Wait, I need help too?

In her first year with us, K had two suicide attempts, two psychiatric hospitalizations, and stays in three different residential mental health treatment facilities for more than six months. In ONE YEAR.

Mind you, this all took place while I was also raising our three little kids and K's little sister, ages two, five, six and seven. It was a LOT.

Within six months of K and her little sister coming into our home, I recognized that I was depressed. Not sad, but depressed—not functioning well, sleeping and eating too much, and extremely cranky, bordering on mean at times *(this does not make me look good, but what is the point of writing this book for you and not being honest?)*. Thankfully, my physician had no problem prescribing an antidepressant, and after a few months I began to feel better.

But you know what I have only just realized? That physician NEVER recommended that I get specific mental health treatment, or heard what I was going through and said, "Tara, get your booty in to see a therapist, this is too much!" In fact, at no point have **any** of my medical doctors made that recommendation, even though I am an open book and have been quite forthcoming about the stresses of being sandwiched between raising suicidal kids and dealing with my aging parents' significant and long-lasting health problems, and then, their deaths. *(I have always thought that the phrase The Sandwich Generation sounded so much more lovely than it actually is. I mean, a sandwich, that sounds fun, like we're going on a picnic . . . not so much. More like being stuck in a freaking panini press. But I digress.)* Suggesting that I consider getting therapy seems like it would have been a real obvious suggestion to make, and I'm more than a bit frustrated that none of them ever did.

I would have two or three discreet seasons of depression in the years to follow, all based on the stress, fear, and sadness of parenting a suicidal teen.

Now, many years later, as I've walked alongside my own child through her suicidal depression, those same feelings have manifested as anxiety. For me, that has looked like trouble sleeping; intrusive, spinning thoughts; an inability to focus; sudden awakening from a dead sleep in a panic attack, with overwhelming dread; a racing heartbeat and racing breathing that can take a looooong time to get under control.

This anxiety has been an entirely new *(and highly unpleasant, might I add)* experience for me, as I've never been one to even worry about things much. As uncomfortable as it is, I guess the only consolation is that it makes perfect sense. My nervous system has been on high alert for much of the last fifteen years, under ridiculous levels of stress, and the human body can only take so much.

None of us will be the special one to escape the laws of biology because we gritted our teeth, pushed through, or toughed it out. Not gonna happen.

Not for me, not for you.

This new anxiety did not respond to any of my own tips and tricks, and I also realized it was beginning to seriously threaten my relationship with A, as I was attempting to manage my fear and anxiety through control and micromanaging.

Maybe you will also find yourself in a place where you realize that your micromanaging is hurting and not helping. Maybe you will find yourself super irritable, or weepy at the grocery store and at work multiple times a week, or overeating, or not eating, or never sleeping, or wanting to do nothing but sleep.

Somehow, you may realize as I have that you need to let your child begin to trust themselves, while you put your trust in God or science or fate or whatever floats your boat, while you also learn to trust your child. And sometimes, you just plain old need more help. Professional help.

In the last two years, I have finally begun seeing my own therapist. I'm not going to lie—I wasn't convinced how helpful it would be at first. I was somewhat skeptical, EVEN THOUGH I have long advocated for people in my situation to get the help of a therapist on this journey. *(Yes, I'm a hypocrite, but at least I own it.)* How could just talking about my stress and anxiety possibly help? I already have a supportive husband and supportive friends; how could therapy be different?

I'm still not sure I understand the magic, but it IS different, and it's been exceedingly helpful.

My therapist has given me new ideas to try regarding specific anxiety symptoms, and she has an extensive background treating first responders and trauma that I actually think was perfect for me. But she also provides a safe place for me to talk about the ongoing issues I'm facing, a place where I can say even my worst thoughts and fears out loud, the ones I wouldn't even share with my husband or my best girlfriends because I wouldn't want to burden, scare or offend them. THAT HAS BEEN KEY FOR ME. Apparently, I have a lot of those thoughts and fears, and I've been protecting everyone else from them. Therapy has been far more helpful than I had imagined it might be, and I definitely wish I'd done it for myself much earlier. In fact, I feel a bit silly for NOT having done it earlier. It's made me a better mom to my, sometimes, suicidal kid, a better wife, and a better mom to my other kids. It has also made me more able to focus on my business productively, including writing this book.

That's why I feel perfectly fine being forceful and bossy and telling YOU that you should consider getting a therapist. I feel like ALL parents of kids who are diagnosed with anything other than the mildest forms of mental health issues should automatically be handed a number to call to arrange for their own therapeutic support, and the fact it isn't standard practice makes no sense to me.

Literally no parent who needs this book, NOT ONE, should be without a therapist. That is personal opinion, that is highly unscientific, and I stand by it. No, not even you, even though you are very special and strong, and you don't have time. Honest. It will help.

Get a therapist.

If you DON'T get the help you need

If you don't get the support you need, you may put your child at greater risk. Maybe dangerously greater risk. Why?

If you are married or have a partner, and one of you is not getting the support you need, it is likely that untreated and unaddressed emotions of anxiety, grief, and anger will come out in the general direction of the other partner. Your relationship will suffer; therefore, your ability to support your child will suffer. Your child will pick up on your relationship stress and make them reluctant to come to either of you for support, because they will want to avoid possibly adding to the tension they feel between you.

Similarly, if you or your partner aren't getting the support you need, your fear and anxiety will lead you to look to your child for reassurance, and they will sense that, and they will not be open and honest with you. Instead, they will hide their scary suicidal thoughts and plans from you to protect you.

As we discussed in the chapter on communication, it is SO tempting to make it about our own feelings. We don't do it on purpose, we don't do it because we're selfish or because we're bad parents. We do it because it's normal. In fact, it's insidious, and nearly impossible to prevent without tremendous intentional effort, and without outside support for our very legitimate emotions.

Get a therapist, join a support group, whatever it takes. Taking care of yourself is MANDATORY if you want to do your best for your child.

When you have a suicidal child, you are experiencing a family emergency, and that's how you should treat it. If your child is in the hospital, or just home from the hospital, it's okay (*and as an advocate I would even say healthy*) to tell family, friends and neighbors that your child is in the middle of a serious mental health crisis. There is no shame in a mental health crisis.

THERE IS NO SHAME IN A MENTAL HEALTH CRISIS.

You cannot do this alone. You cannot do this just with your spouse or partner, if you are so lucky to have one. Parenting a child who struggles with suicidal ideation is just too difficult, and if you don't already have a strong circle of support in your life, your own village, you need to create it NOW.

In addition to a great therapist with whom you click, you need friends who will listen, you need other parents who have been through or are going through a similar journey, you need experts who will support you, and you need spiritual mentors or leaders who will pray for you if that's important in your life.

If you don't happen to have such a circle of support set up already, being told you must go create one is probably not a message you want to hear. You are already pretty booked up, what with parenting a child who has suicidal thoughts and all. I know, and I feel a little guilty for telling you to go do it anyway.

But go do it anyway.

Parenting through mental illness is simply too exhausting, too difficult, too likely to challenge your faith in yourself and in your parenting, for you to go this alone.

On the one hand, when your child is suicidal, it is a full-out life-threatening emergency in which your child's life is literally at stake.

On the other hand, it is also an ongoing situation, and you can't operate at 110% for very long at all.

• • • • • • •

But first, let me tell you this: do not hesitate to tell people how they can help. When people find out what your family is going through, they are going to want to help because they care about you. Sure, they may be a little more awkward about it because the crisis is related to mental health, which still makes people weird and awkward in our society, but they will want to help.

IT IS OK TO ASK FOR HELP.

IT IS OK TO ACCEPT HELP.

IT IS OK TO BE SPECIFIC ABOUT WHAT IS HELPFUL.

Doing so will actually help your friends and family because they don't want to be extra trouble or work, and they care; they just may need some pointers.

Because we are all often well-intentioned, but particularly in a situation involving serious mental health issues, we're still not very good at knowing what to do or how to react or how to help. So although you shouldn't have to be responsible for helping your community know how to help, the reality is that if you want help that is actually helpful, you need to tell folks what you need.

**IT IS OK TO ASK FOR HELP. IT IS OK TO ACCEPT HELP.
IT IS OK TO BE SPECIFIC ABOUT WHAT IS HELPFUL.**

Also: you cannot do this alone. You need a village.

Finally, remember, as always, you have my full permission to say NO to the following "helpful" type of offers: any and all advice you did not request!

"Oh, thank you for caring about us enough to share how your aunt Gertrude cured her depression and OCD with apple cider vinegar and crystals. Thankfully, we have a great team of experts and a plan for LisaSueJo, but I appreciate the thought. Bless your heart . . . *(execute internal eye roll.)*"

WHAT TO SAY WHEN SOMEONE SAYS, "IF THERE'S ANYTHING WE CAN DO, JUST ASK."

I've made it easy and given you some options. Here are some ideas you can have at the ready when someone says the inevitable: "if there's anything we can do, just ask." *(Of course, you will meter these requests out proportionally according to your relationship with the individual. Probably best not to ask the dentist if she'd swing by and water the garden. Unless she's your dentist and your sister, then she should definitely pick up a hose.)* So, when someone asks what they could do, choose from and adapt one of the following if nothing comes to mind.

- Actually, I'd love it if you'd just let me ramble, and tell you what's happening, and tell you how scared I am. I just need you to listen.

- Yes, you could bring a dinner this week. We love anything pasta and we hate mushrooms and fish. *(Or whatever is true for you, obviously.)(Yes, you really can say that. It's okay. No one wants a mushroom fish casserole. Speak up for yourself.)*

- Yes, you could organize our friends to bring us some dinners for the next couple of weeks; we love anything pasta and we hate mushrooms and fish. *(Or whatever is true for you, obviously.)*

- Well, it would be a big help if you could get little Jimmy to and from soccer practice on Wednesday for a couple of weeks because we have a therapy appointment those afternoons.

- I've got to be at the hospital all afternoon Wednesday for psychiatrist appointments, could you please have Landon over for a play date?

CONTINUED ➡

- *(For really good friends, or your mom, or your mother-in-law)* Oh, my goodness, we are completely out of clean clothes. I'd be so grateful if you could do a couple of loads of laundry for us. Start with towels and underwear, please?

- Are you going to be running to Costco this week by any chance? We're almost out of toilet paper, and I need milk, bananas and NINE BOXES OF HAAGEN DAZ ICE CREAM BARS, that would be swell. What's that? Am I particularly stressed out, why ever do you ask?

- I really need to get myself a therapist, any chance you could ask around for recommendations?

- Our dishwasher is broken, and I'd love it if someone could look up the numbers of a few repair places I could call. Even better, would you call them?

- Pray. Just pray for us.

- Could you take the other kids to the movies this week?

- Could you hang out and sit with my teen this afternoon so I can take a nap/go for a walk/browse the aisles at Sephora because I just need to be normal for five minutes?

Don't roll your eyes at me

I repeat. None of us will be the special one to escape the laws of biology because we gritted our teeth, pushed through, or toughed it out. Not gonna happen.

You are not just having a difficult emotional journey. The stress and trauma of parenting a suicidal child is a physical, biological experience, and the physical effects are not optional, nor are they escapable. They are manageable, though, if you are intentional about your self-care.

Unmanaged? Chronic high stress such as what we experience in this journey, can deplete your immune system function; increase systemic inflammation in your body; cause mental health issues such as depression, anxiety and PTSD; and increase the risk of a host of other illnesses, ranging from heart disease to GI issues.

Part of being effective and intentional with your self-care is realizing that the coping skills required for the standard temporary stresses of your previous "normal" life are what we might call Beginner Level Self-Care Skills, or as your kids would say, Mid Self-Care Skills; you are in need of Master Level Self-Care Skills.

The Boring Four

Building Master Level Self-Care Skills starts with what I call the **Boring Four—sleep, nutrition, exercise, community.**

Sleep. Nutrition. Exercise. Community. See, I told you it was boring!

When it comes to taking care of ourselves and practicing good, intentional and effective self-care, the lowest hanging fruit, not surprisingly, comes from focusing on and sticking to consistent routines of basic, boring practices that we all know reduce stress and anxiety, but we all also ignore at will:

Sleep—I'm not going to mince words here. You need to stop lying to yourself about how little sleep you need. People humble-bragging that they only need four to five hours of sleep a night has become the new "oh, gosh, I'm just SO busy." NOPE. You know what percentage of people can REALLY get away with four to five hours of sleep a night? 1-2%. That's it. Is it possible this includes you? Sure. Is it likely? No. ESPECIALLY not while parenting a child struggling with suicidal thoughts.

Brains heal and take out the garbage while we sleep, and if they don't get a chance to take out the garbage, science is making it increasingly clear that bad things happen in our brains.

Sleep is my personal kryptonite. I have learned that I absolutely cannot mess with this. Any other 9-10-hours-of-sleep-a-night-needed folks? I had to adopt some pretty counter-cultural practices to honor what my body and brain required, and the stress and chaos I was experiencing. From the time my kids were in middle school, they were often getting up, getting their own breakfast, and leaving to walk to school or the bus without me. *(Bonus, I had children who were and ARE capable of getting their own breakfast and getting themselves out the door on time with all of their belongings. Most of the time. It's amazing what our kids are capable of when we expect things from them.)* Even now, my normal workday starts at 10 a.m. Either I get enough sleep, or everything goes to crap. I've learned that, and I don't mess with it.

Nutrition, eating well—includes hydration! We all know this is important, and this isn't my area of expertise. Many others are more qualified than I am to help with nutrition. What I will say is that there is a quickly growing body of science that points to the critical connection between our gut and our brains, and how well they function. Even on the difficult days, the hard days, the chaotic impossible days, try to do what you can to focus on nurturing your body with quality food, including protein and fiber, that will fuel you. Also, stay hydrated, as dehydration has surprisingly powerful effects on our energy, mood and even decision making.

Exercise/nature—exercise has measurable powerful antidepressive and stress-relieving effects. What's important here is to figure out what works for you, what type of movement is most effective and helpful for you. For me, sometimes it's vigorous *Beat Saber* sessions on my kids' virtual reality goggles, or dance exercise videos in my kitchen, or longs walks in nature. High intensity exercise releases endorphins. This isn't about weight loss; this is about embracing regular movement that feels good, dare I even say feels fun. Which is why I will never have the same self-care routines as my friends who tell me about how running is so critical to their own mental health. Blech. I don't run unless a bear is chasing me. Even then, if I'm with a friend who can run faster, I'll probably just give up.

Exposure to nature has a powerful effect on our brains and our spirits. We are powerfully wired to experience nature, and we need it. Whenever you can, go outside. Breathe in the air, look around, notice the leaves, listen to the birds. Don't overcomplicate this. It doesn't have to be an overnight backpacking trip. One study found that even listening to a short clip of less than six minutes of birdsong reduced symptoms of anxiety and depression and improved moods.

Community—Stay connected with friends and family. This also helps build emotional resiliency so you can support one another. Again, if you don't have people, get some! If you don't have people, get brave and go find and build your support network. If you're struggling, sometimes just telling someone can bring meaningful relief. AND it opens the door for them to share if they are having a similar experience. Short on community? That's another good reason to get your own therapist, as a helpful measure to get you through while you intentionally build community.

· · · · · · ·

Right now, you may be frustrated with me. "Listen, woman, have you forgotten who you are writing to? Tara, we're a LITTLE BUSY at the moment, what with our suicidal child and all." I get it, I promise. I also know that if you completely ignore the Boring Four, YOU WILL NOT BE THE PARENT YOUR CHILD NEEDS RIGHT NOW. You don't have to be perfect. Right now is not the time to put pressure on yourself to develop a five days a week exercise routine at the gym, and also meal plan on Sundays so you're cooking homemade meals with organic ingredients every night except for the nights you are backpacking with your close friends in nature.

Heck no, that's not what I'm advocating. I'm just saying, do the best you can in these four areas. Don't ignore them. Pick a baby step in one or two areas to start with. Drink more water every day, and get eight hours of sleep most nights. Or take a break at lunch and go for a 10-minute walk while you connect with a friend on the phone. Baby steps.

Parent PTSD is real

Gonna get really real for a few paragraphs, maybe skip ahead if you're feeling fragile.

But if not, and especially if you're still feeling like ignoring your wellbeing is a workable option, or feeling defensive about your lack of self-care, keep reading. PTSD due to parenting a child with a serious mental illness, particularly a suicidal child, is a real thing. Just the knowledge that your child does not want to be alive is something your brain can barely wrap itself around, and just that knowledge alone, not to mention the fear that comes with it, is trauma. Real, legit, trauma.

Being with your child after a significant self-harm episode or a suicide attempt is horrifying, heartbreaking trauma. Sitting in a room in an emergency room, as I have, listening to your child tell the doctor that they are tired of trying, tired of feeling hopeless, and that the only reason they haven't killed themselves is that they haven't figured out how to do it so you or another family member doesn't find them, is horrifying, heartbreaking trauma.

Trauma that can cause physical symptoms, emotional symptoms; trauma that may need medical (psychological—remember, brains are an organ and brain care is medical care) attention if it is too severe, too prolonged or if it begins to interfere with your day-to-day life.

Honestly, just contemplating losing your child to suicide is horrifying, heartbreaking trauma, and not trauma that you should walk through alone. Full stop. Whether it's too much for your friends and family to walk through with you, I can't tell you, but it may be. Don't do this alone. Don't do this while ignoring your own self-care. It's too much, it's too hard, and you deserve better.

YOU AIN'T GOT TIME FOR THAT! THINGS YOU HAVE PERMISSION NOT TO DO RIGHT NOW

- Care about housecleaning—do what you can, what is required for health and hygiene purposes, and ignore the rest.

- Engage in small talk—it's exhausting, does not renew your energy but actually depletes it, and you don't have the emotional bandwidth. Focus right now on more meaningful connections with friends and family. Aggressively avoid situations and events that will unnecessarily suck the remaining energy from your body. *(If it works for you, you can definitely assign a good friend or family member to be the go-between who tells folks what is going on so you don't have to.)*

- Worry about your child's school, credits, or grades. This is really hard, I know. But the most important thing is getting your child healthy. School will always be there, they can and will catch up when they are ready. Honest.

- Have it all together. You don't, and you can't, and that's okay. You'll get there when you can.

Planning for yourself, post-crisis

You should plan on losing a few days for every crisis, and not being able to function. I wish someone had told me earlier in this journey that after every serious episode, every suicide attempt, major depressive episode with suicidal ideation, serious self-harm or other mental health crisis, that I would need to just write off the next few days. Instead, just as an episode was ending, and life was returning to "normal," I would then dive in and try to make up for the work projects that had been missed, the housework that hadn't happened, the missed laundry, and whatever else had been put on hold in the moment.

Except I couldn't. Every time, I would wind up beating myself up because I couldn't get anything done. I just seemed to wander around the house, stare into space, or ineffectually start and then not finish a task. Every time.

I finally realized that this post-episode funk was not optional. It was part of how my mind and body needed to handle and recover from the emergency, and that I needed to just schedule it into my mental, and even actual, calendar.

I found the same requirements applied, by the way, when caring for my elderly mother, who was in tenuous poor health for the last several years of her life. Every serious fall, every trip to the hospital, each new onset of illness, each major health event led to a few days afterward of me not being able to do anything.

This is frustrating, I get it. Because when these crises happen, out of necessity we DO have to set things aside, put them on hold, let the house go. When the crisis is over, we feel obliged to jump back in and make up for it.

Here's what you need to understand: *there is a physical cost to the emotional energy you muster and expend in each crisis. That cost is not optional. It will be paid, one way or another.* Fear, anxiety, extreme hypervigilance, and grief are certainly emotional experiences, but they are also physically exhausting. They are not "just" emotional experiences, but are also physical experiences, driven by very real biological processes such as adrenaline surges, and your body will need time to rest and recover.

Could you just try and power through, ignore the impact of the experience you've just had, and push forward? Yes, you could. If you do, then I promise you will eventually find yourself overly exhausted, getting sick, sacrificing your own mental health, and thus even less able to complete the tasks of life AND to support your child. And first? First, you'll get really cranky. Or uncontrollably weepy. Truth. I don't recommend it.

If your child's mental health has led to you finding this book, then you are most likely not in a sprint. This situation is unlikely to be one bad episode and then everything will be fine. I'm so sorry, but that's true. You need to think of parenting a child with mental illness not as a sprint, but as a marathon.

Therefore, as a crisis episode comes to an end, just make a note to yourself. "Okay, now I need two or three days to recover, during which I will have no expectations for getting anything done other than resting. If I manage anything else, that will be fine, but I will not beat myself up if I don't."

Focus on the basics—extra sleep, nutrition that is fueling and healing, a walk outside, read, watch ridiculous movies, whatever will rest your mind, soul and body. Connect with your support circle, friends and family, spiritual leaders, whomever has YOUR back while you are busy having your child's back.

If you accept reality and give yourself an intentional break, two to three days to focus on self-care and rest, you will be most able to THEN return to the tasks of work and home, as well as managing your child's care.

Conclusion

You're a good parent. Know how I know? Because you've read this book, a book you NEVER thought you would ever read when you brought home that sweet baby from the hospital or brought this child into your home.

No one WANTS to read this book, not really. The fact you are reading it, that you've picked it up and chosen to spend time with it, means you want the best for your child. You want to be YOUR best for your child during this impossible season.

Way to go, Mom.

Way to go, Dad.

Way to go, Grandma or Grandpa, Auntie or Uncle.

• • • • • • •

Whoever you are to this child you care about, thank you for walking alongside them, for caring for them, and for wanting the best possible life for them.

Because of you, they have more support, more resources, and more hope.

Way to go.

K and A, today

Throughout this book, I've shared some difficult stories with you about my niece, K, and my daughter, A. I don't want to leave you with those stories as the end, because they aren't.

Let me circle back to where my mental health parenting journey started, with K. K spent several years after she came to us revolving through residential mental health treatment, psychiatric hospital admissions, stays in our home and in therapeutic foster care, and a few different alternative schools. There were multiple suicide attempts, SO MUCH therapy, and a lot of hard work by both K and us. There were also significant stretches of time during which we were tempted to lose hope, not sure K was going to be able to rise above her trauma, PTSD, depression and anxiety, and survive.

But after years of other people believing in her, loving her, holding her accountable, and providing her with compassion and support, K finally began to believe in herself.

I'm ridiculously, obnoxiously proud to share that K eventually graduated high school with a full unmodified diploma. She plans to go to college, and she's a certified peer wellness specialist, ready to support others on their mental health journey.

Today, she is a young married mom with three little ones she adores and mothers well. Not only that, but as I write this, she has become a foster mom herself, taking in two more little family members to nurture and love.

She's not all better, and she may never be completely free of PTSD, depression, and anxiety. She still sometimes experiences mental health symptoms and hard days. But she also has the tools now to manage those symptoms; she knows when she needs to check in with a psychiatrist or see her therapist more often; and she is an effective, proactive advocate for herself and her family. She has a meaningful, mostly happy life with a lot of hope for the future.

What about my daughter? Well, A tried college for a semester and realized she wasn't ready, and she wasn't healthy enough. She lived with friends for a bit, and then moved home to really focus on figuring out her mental health, connecting with a new psychiatric nurse practitioner for treatment and therapy, and learning to understand and live with her depression, her ADHD, and her autism. She has committed to doing the work, even though it isn't easy and the path isn't clear, even though she still has days when her brain lies to her, and she feels like the world is crashing down around her. I'm ridiculously proud of her for getting up every day, choosing herself and choosing life.

A is beautiful, funny, creative and smart, and as much as I hate her mental health struggles and wish she did not have them, I also know that it's part of her journey, and that on the other side she will be stronger for having been through it.

K and A may always live with at least the occasional suicidal thought, and they may always be at higher risk. I have no guarantees that K or A will always do as well as they are right now.

But I have no guarantees that I won't be hit by a bus tomorrow, either.

I've learned that life is precious, and even when it's scary, we have to grab every moment of joy, and turn our backs on the fear as much as we can.

We have to stay present, communicate openly, advocate fiercely, and take care of ourselves.

We have to love our kids, the best we can.

Remember to hope

Can I tell you something? Someday, you will be able to breathe easy, or easier, again. You will be able to sleep without jumping at every noise, you will stop checking their location on your phone, and you will be able to relax.

You may not believe it now, but someday you will have enough distance from this experience to help another parent. You will share your story one day, either privately over coffee or even to a group, and your vulnerability will unlock someone else's courage to reach out and get the help they need, or to get help for their child.

You will feel a particularly tender depth of gratitude on the good days, and it will feel suspiciously like hope. You will want to back away, not look directly at it. But do it. Look it directly, full in the face, because it will be real, it will be true in that moment, and that very real hope will deserve to be the center of your attention far more than any of the fears vying to pull your attention away.

There will be many points of uncertainty along the way, moments when we may have to relinquish our child to the care of someone else who can reach them better than we can, or help them heal better than we can.

But this is just a deeper and more intense version of what is already inherent to the parenting process, isn't it? In letting them go, maybe even into the care of others who can guide them and treat them in ways we can't, we do the important work of giving them the dignity of their own path, and the ability to begin creating their own recovery. Those are lessons that will make our children stronger, more resilient, and more compassionate human beings long after their suicidal thoughts have faded, become tolerable, or even gone away.

In the meantime, we are learning more and more all the time about effective treatments and approaches to help people who live with mental health issues and suicidal thoughts. Most people who live with suicidal thoughts, or even attempt to die by suicide, do not die by suicide. It is hard to cling to these hopeful truths when it feels so dark and scary in the moment of a crisis, or in the ongoing exhaustion of crises, but they are still true.

Hang in there, Mama. Hang in there, Dad. Don't give up, Grandpa, or Auntie, or foster parent. There is hope. No one knows this child like you do, no one loves them like you do. With you by their side, they will know you love them and they can begin to heal.

Hang in there. Hold on to hope for your child, until they can hope for themselves.

Me? I'm holding on to hope for you, for those moments when you can't find it or grab onto it. I believe in you. You can do this.

Appendix: Additional Resources

Strategies to try with your kid in the immediate moment

In an escalated moment, when your child is overwhelmed by big emotions, when they cannot access any coping skills, or when you both need a break, these strategies may prove helpful.

Create a calming kit on their phone with images, music, readings, videos, reminders of smells and touches that they like.

5 senses exercise:

- Name 5 things you see
- Name 4 things you can touch
- Name 3 things you can hear
- Name 2 things you can taste
- Name 1 thing you can smell

Three Technique:

- Draw a triangle on your hand
- Name 3 things you can see, hear, and touch
- Breathe in for a count of 3, hold for 3, breath out for 3
- Remember your 3 people/places that make you feel safe
- Clench and unclench muscles 3 times

Opposite Action

- Try the opposite action exercise—make it a challenge or a game, particularly with younger kids. For example:
- Feeling sad? Watch something funny.
- Is your current emotion anger, and you want to yell? Try whispering.

Practice the STOP technique:

- **S**top
- **T**ake a breath
- **O**bserve—internally and externally. What's going on?
- **P**roceed—make an intentional decision based on your observations

Call or text with a trusted person: a family member, friend, coach, youth leader.

An Incredibly Subjective and Incomplete List of Other Resources That Might Help

Websites

988lifeline.org – National Suicide Prevention Lifeline. Text option also available at Crisis Text Line (specifically youth focused), text 'TALK' to 741741 to speak or text with a trained counselor.

NAMI.org – the National Alliance on Mental Illness. NAMI has local chapters around the U.S. that offer free, evidence-based education and training. Often, they also offer support groups for parents and caregivers.

mhanational.org – Mental Health America, another great nonprofit dedicated to the promotion of mental health, well-being, and condition prevention.

twloha.com – To Write Love on Her Arms, focused on suicide and self-injury

thetrevorproject.org – The Trevor Project, specialized support, crisis services and advocacy for LGBTQ+ young people, including 24/7 chat, text and phone crisis counselors

afsp.org – American Foundation for Suicide Prevention

johnnysambassadors.org – Johnny's Ambassadors has great information on marijuana, young people, and mental health. *Trigger warning:* started by a mom who lost a child to suicide as a result of cannabis psychosis.

Books:

Anything written by Julie A. Fast, an expert on bipolar disorder and schizophrenia who has published several books, including books for family members. Her website and Facebook groups for family members are also tremendously helpful for anyone with a loved one who lives with serious mental illness. Her books include ***Loving Someone with Bipolar Disorder*** and ***Take Charge of Bipolar Disorder***. Her website and links to extensive online articles can be found at: https://juliefast.com/

We've Got This: Journal for Parenting Kids with Mental Health Struggles, Tara Rolstad (Amazon); A tracking journal for behaviors, symptoms, appointments and medications, as well as space for you to record your experiences.

OMG That's Me! 3: Bipolar Disorder, Depression, PTSD, Mental Health and Humor, Dave Mowry and Tara Rolstad (Amazon); A fun and inspiring book telling the stories of how six people used stand-up comedy to transform their experience with mental illness and their lives.

You Are Not Alone, the NAMI Guide to Navigating Mental Health with Advice from Experts and Wisdom from Real People and Families, from the National Alliance on Mental Illness (NAMI)

I am Not Sick, I Don't Need Help! How to Help Someone Accept Treatment, Xavier Amador (all major booksellers); written primarily about schizophrenia, but immensely helpful for many people who love someone with serious mental illness, including bipolar disorder and addiction, especially in situations in which lack of insight is a symptom of the disorder.

Hope for Troubled Minds: Tributes to Those with Brain Illnesses and Their Loved Ones, Tony Roberts; Amazon; a trove of tributes, collected to celebrate the lives, legacy, and strength of those who lead brave lives in the face of brain disorders and mental illness.

If your child is experiencing serious mental illness, including psychotic spectrum disorders such as schizophrenia or schizoaffective disorder:

TAC.org – the Treatment Advocacy Center provides advocacy, public education, and support for individuals and families affected by SMI, including a helpline and resource center.

The TAC Helpline provides individualized support for individuals and caregivers navigating the complex SMI system: https://www .tac.org/helpline/

The TAC Joan C. Scott Community Resource Center provides information, resources, and support for those seeking help for someone affected by severe mental illness: https://www.tac.org /community-resource-center/

Check out these TAC articles specifically:

- Psychosis: https://www.tac.org/resources/first-episode
  -psychosis/ and https://www.tac.org/resources/psychosis/

- Safety planning: https://www.tac.org/resources/violence
  -and-safety-plans/

- Communication tips: https://www.tac.org/resources/
  communication-tips/

- Emergencies: https://www.tac.org/resources/emergencies/

Also:

- University of Washington SPIRIT Center: https://
  uwspiritcenter.org/family-caregiver-support-programs/

- LEAP Institute, based on the work of Dr. Xavier Amador:
  https://leapinstitute.org/

- Julie Fast: https://juliefast.com/

Working with the school

https://www.nami.org/your-journey/kids-teens-and-young-adults/kids
  /getting-your-child-mental-health-support-and-accommodations
  -in-school/

If your child is an adult with SMI

Consider talking with them about completing a Psychiatric Advance
Directive when they are stable and not in crisis. This document,
provided to the team upon admission, can help ensure your child's
needs and wishes are respected during a crisis, especially if it
involves hospitalization, voluntary or involuntary.

For more information: https://www.tac.org/resources/pad/

Random other helpful web pages

For hope and stories of recovery:
    https://988lifeline.org/stories/

Removing lethal means:
    https://www.sprc.org/sites/default/files/Handout-WhatClients
    OrFamilies.pdf

Safety Plan template: https://docs.google.com/document/d/101So
    GPZAnbagQCHr-v3epRLOmeHaidoPft1RBK27-EI/edit

To get a gun safety kit: https://projectchildsafe.org/get-a-safety-kit/

Apps that may be helpful

Full disclosure, I've never been able to get my own child to try any of
    these, but OTHER people have found them helpful:

Not OK – recommended for safety planning, developed by young
    adults who have lived with suicidality.

Cope Notes

Headspace

Insight Timer

Calm

Smiling Mind App

Acknowledgements

The first and most obvious people to thank for this book are the young people in my life who have experienced suicidal thinking—my niece, K, her sisters, and my daughter A. I will never be able to express my gratitude, pride, and admiration for the courage you've shown to get up every day when you were feeling hopeless, when you didn't see a way forward, or believe there was a reason to keep trying. Thank you. Thank you for doing the work; thank you for allowing us to believe in you until you could believe in the hope of your own future; thank you for everything you've taught me; and thank you for forgiving all my dumb mistakes. I'm a better parent, aunt, and human because of each of you. Don't stop, keep going. You are so deeply loved, and we need you here. I am not complete without you.

· · · · · · ·

This book was a surprise to me, born at a writer's retreat where I had intended to work on an upcoming speech for my professional speaking business after a difficult few weeks supporting my daughter. I sat down to work the first morning, and instead of my new speech, the first several pages of this book poured out.

I was not pleased. Nope, I was freaked out. I did not want to write this book. It scared me and felt overwhelming. In fact, God and I had a long argument about it that weekend, with a lot of whining and protesting on my end. He won. I am grateful He did, and grateful for His love and work in my life.

That retreat was The Writer's Advance, run by my friend and mentor Marc Schelske. I'm deeply grateful to Marc, and to one of the coaches that weekend, Paul Pastor, and to all of the participants at the Writer's Advance who have cheered me on.

Just as it takes a village to raise a child, it takes a village to write a book. So many others have contributed to this work, either through their professional wisdom or personal support, and each was integral to the final outcome.

Too often, we hesitate to do big, bold, necessary things because of our litigious society, and indeed, without those types of concerns I think more resources such as this would exist. But this book did need the requisite legal disclaimers, and I am grateful to Bob Cumbow, attorney and partner at Miller Nash, who was generous, kind and wise as he helped me think all of that through.

· · · · · · ·

Early interviews and conversations with these folks helped me form the right questions as I began to flesh out the project: Jill Baker, LSC, Youth Suicide Prevention Coordinator with the Oregon Health Authority; Galli Murray, LCSW, Suicide Prevention Coordinator with Clackamas County, Oregon; Angie Welty, author of *"Mayday: a Mother's Story of Hope After Nearly Losing Her Son to Suicide"*; and Crystal Larson, LCW, MSCW, Lines for Life, Oregon.

I'm also grateful for a long, insightful and encouraging conversation with Jonathan Singer, Ph.D, LCSW, and Past President of the American Association of Suicidology.

As writing was wrapping up, I accidentally and serendipitously found a suicide researchers' listserv online. Several members of that group responded to my out-of-the-blue request to review the manuscript with generosity, wisdom and encouragement: Wendy Sefcik, Co-Chair, New Jersey Youth Suicide Prevention Advisory Council; Inga Giske, DNP, PMHNP-BC, Consultation Liaison Psychiatry; COL(Ret) George D. Patrin, M.D., MHA, CEO of the Serendipity Alliance; Elizabeth McErlean, LCSW, LISW; Tammy Tucker, Psy.D., FACHE; and (with extra gratitude for an especially long, generous Zoom call) Jerri Carr with the Treatment Advocacy Center.

ACKNOWLEDGEMENTS

A project like this requires significant technical support, and I've been blessed with fantastic partners. Thank you to my wise editor and friend, Leanne, who is always right about punctuation but, more importantly, is an amazing guide to the deep work of shaping a book. From my earliest days in this space, you have been a trusted resource and friend. You have shaped my writing, my advocacy, and my approach to parenting, and this is only our second book together!

As a creative author and professional speaker with self-diagnosed (but let's be honest, pretty obvious) ADHD and a LOT going on in my life, I consider the hiring of my business coach, Retha Nichole, to be one of my wisest decisions ever. Retha cheers me on and keeps me moving forward instead of spinning or spiraling. So glad you're in my life!

I am also grateful to my creative and speedy graphic designer Julie Lucas; my audiobook producer, Ralph Scott, and the team at Squeaky Cheese Productions; and to interior designer and founder of Printed Page Studios, Rachel Valliere.

I have learned so much from my brilliant friend, author and serious mental illness expert Julie Fast. So much of what I know and understand about bipolar disorder, schizophrenia, psychosis, and loving people with those illnesses I owe to Julie, and the world is better because of your research, your books and your support of that community. We've spent so many hours together, working over chips and guac, laughing about movies we don't agree on, and mutually preaching to the choir on all the ways our system needs to do better for individuals and families with mental illness. Thank you for sharing your brilliance and thank you for being my friend.

To my tiny Facebook group of other parents of kids who've been suicidal: Kati, Andrea, Nichole, Amelia, Charlotte, Heidi, Jennifer and Leigh Ann, thank you. Thank you for raising your hand, for not letting me feel alone, for brainstorming ideas, reading early versions, voting on covers, and not making fun of me when I ignored you for months on end when life got too real and I had to step away and take a break.

To every parent, caregiver, or family member who has shared their story with me, asked for my advice, let me cry with you and pray for

145

you, thank you. In some way, each of your stories and struggles shaped this book.

To every therapist, psychiatric nurse practitioner, psychiatrist, emergency room provider, nurse, treatment center staff, and skills trainer who has poured into my young people in all of their tough moments, and in to the lives of countless others, thank you. Thank you for doing difficult, lifesaving work that changes people's futures; and thank you for doing it for far too little money or recognition. You should ALL be making Taylor Swift money.

I am forever grateful to my fellow professional speaker friends and colleagues, especially Lauren, and my NSA Oregon community.

To Carolyn, my own therapist (yay, therapy for us parents!), who I hope forgives me for occasionally asking, "So, what is it we're really doing here, again?" Thank you for helping me value my own experience, my own emotions, and my own healing; and for giving me a place to say the hard and scary things.

I categorically, unquestionably would not have made it without dear friends who encouraged me, sat with me while I cried, listened to the latest crisis of the day, celebrated the little wins and the big successes, prayed for me, called me out when I needed it, and loved me. Some of you were there every week for small group, or you lived across the street, or you were there back in the early parenting days on the playground at pickup. One of you was present at the birth of each of my children, and one of you I've known since we were both infants. To Julie, Karen, Barbara; Kati, Ingrid, Paige, and Cindy; Kathy, Holly and Mary; Libby and Susan; and so many more, thank you. You have all given me support, strength, courage and comfort, and you are all my sisters.

I'm grateful to my parents, Howard and Carol, who, though they are no longer with us, showed me how to show up for my people, and how to love. I am a powerful communicator because of my dad, and I owe my delightful squeaky wheel superpowers to my mom, who could write a letter to the editor like no one else.

I'm so grateful for my three kids, who are kind, good, smart people who make me laugh and who I know will make this world a better place.

I love you, I'm proud to be your mom, and I hope that whatever you've lost from me when I was helping someone else, you've gotten back in some other way.

To my husband David, thank you for your constant support, for saying yes to all my crazy ideas, for killing the spiders, and for doing math for me. You are my rock, and I could not do any of this without you. I love you.

Kickstarter Backers

The publication of this book was made possible through the support of more than 100 people who stepped forward as Backers of the Kickstarter campaign. I'm deeply grateful to every single one of those Kickstarter Backers, but especially the following:

Michelle Amberg
Suzy Anderson, LPC
Anonymous
Diane and Mike Bays
Libby Boatwright
Josh and Laurel Boverhof
Gwen Bruss
Megan Capper
Catherine Meye Chiba
Jon Colby
Susie Marto Crowell
Richard and Nancy DeBusman
Ellen Falbo
Julie A. Fast
Chuck Hagele
Jennifer Hepler
Ro Hinzdel
Traci Humphrey
Andrea Kelly

Kris Kelso

Sabel Ketler

Lauren Lamb

Ingrid McKinley

Glennis J. McNeal

Cynthia Miguel

Molly

NW Resiliency Project

Rick and Amelia Nys

Bonnie & Jon Peterson

Carolyn Powell

Joyce Pruyn

Rena Rabe

Veronica Riley

Edde Rolstad

Marc Schelske

Susan Schrader

Squeaky Cheese Productions, LLC

Julie Strong

Leanne Sype

Lauren Teague

Whitney Treloar

Julie True

Shayna Vance

Jen and Craig Weber

About the Author

Tara is a professional speaker and mental health advocate with a unique combination of expertise, authenticity, and humor. More importantly, she has parented teens who were suicidal and live with severe mental illness, and she gets it.

Whether in keynotes, on social media, in trainings or at the grocery store, Tara breaks down stigma around mental illness by teaching people how to understand and support individuals who struggle with mental health. In addition to her work as a speaker for corporate and association audiences, she is a program partner with NAMI (National Alliance on Mental Illness) Washington County and NAMI Clackamas County in Oregon, and the founder and director of her own mental health conferences for school districts, faith communities, and other organizations. She is also the author of "We've Got This: Journal for Parenting Kids with Mental Health" and "OMG That's Me! 3: Bipolar Disorder, Depression, PTSD, Mental Health and Humor."

Tara is the proud mom of three kind, brilliant and hysterically funny young adult kids, and proud auntie to her amazing nieces. She lives in a suburb of Portland, Oregon with her husband David, one brilliant cat, and another cat that's... pretty.

Follow Tara on Instagram or LinkedIn, and find out more at her website tararolstad.com.

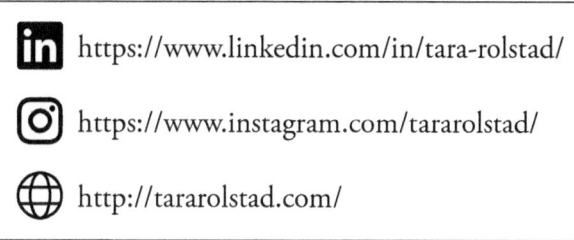

https://www.linkedin.com/in/tara-rolstad/

https://www.instagram.com/tararolstad/

http://tararolstad.com/

www.ingramcontent.com/pod-product-compliance
Lightning Source LLC
Chambersburg PA
CBHW061758120626
46550CB00005B/2040